Occupational Health and Hygiene in Industry

Occupational Health and Hygiene in Industry

SK Haldar
Former Deputy Director General
Directorate General of Factory Advice Service and Labour Institutes
Ministry of Labour and Employment, Government of India
and
Former Deputy Principal Medical Officer
M/s Hindustan Cables Ltd. (Central Government Enterprise), West Bengal, India

CBSPD

CBS Publishers & Distributors Pvt Ltd

New Delhi • Bengaluru • Chennai • Kochi • Kolkata • Lucknow • Mumbai
Gujarat • Hyderabad • Jharkhand • Nagpur • Patna • Pune • Uttarakhand

Disclaimer

Science and technology are constantly changing fields. New research and experience broaden the scope of information and knowledge. The author has tried his best in giving information available to him while preparing the material for this book. Although, all efforts have been made to ensure optimum accuracy of the material, yet it is quite possible some errors might have been left uncorrected. The publisher, the printer and the author will not be held responsible for any inadvertent errors, omissions or inaccuracies.

Occupational Health and Hygiene in Industry

ISBN: 978-93-5466-492-2

First Edition: 2023
Reprint: 2025

Published by Satish Kumar Jain and produced by Varun Jain for
CBS Publishers & Distributors Pvt Ltd
4819/XI Prahlad Street, 24 Ansari Road, Daryaganj, New Delhi 110 002, India.
Ph: 011-23289259, 23266868 Website: www.cbspd.com
e-mail: delhi@cbspd.com

Corporate Office: 204 FIE, Industrial Area, Patparganj, Delhi-110092
Ph: 011-4934 4934 e-mail: publishing@cbspd.com; publicity@cbspd.com

Branches

- **Bengaluru:** Seema House 2975, 17th Cross, K.R. Road, Banasankari 2nd Stage, Bengaluru 560 070, Karnataka
  Ph: +91-80-26771678/79 Fax: +91-80-26771680 e-mail: bangalore@cbspd.com
- **Chennai:** 18/8B, Subbarayan Street, Shenoy Nagar, Chennai 600 030, Tamil Nadu
  Ph: +91-44-42032115, 26681266 e-mail: chennai@cbspd.com
- **Kochi:** 42/1325, 1326, Power House Road, Opp KSEB Power House, Ernakulam 682 018, Kochi, Kerala
  Ph: +91-484-4059061-65 Fax: +91-484-4059065 e-mail: kochi@cbspd.com
- **Kolkata:** 147, Hind Ceramics Compound, 1st Floor, Nilgunj Road, Belghoria, Kolkata 700 056, West Bengal, India
  Ph: +91-033-25633055 e-mail: kolkata@cbspd.com
- **Lucknow:** Basement, Khushnuma Complex, 7-Meerabai Marg (behind Jawahar Bhawan), Lucknow 226 001, UP
  Ph: +91-522-400032 e-mail: tiwari.lucknow@cbspd.com
- **Mumbai:** PWD Shed, Gala no. 25/26, Ramchandra Bhatt Marg, Next to JJ Hospital Gate no. 2
  Opp. Union Bank of India, Noorbaug, Mumbai-400009, Maharashtra, India
  Ph: 022-60061880/89 e-mail: mumbai@cbspd.com

Representatives

- **Gujarat** 0-9879558667
- **Hyderabad** 0-9885175004
- **Jharkhand** 0-9811541605
- **Nagpur** 0-8692091830
- **Patna** 0-9334159340
- **Pune** 0-9664372571
- **Uttarakhand** 0-9716462459

Printed at: Mudrak, Noida, UP, India

Preface

Postgraduate diploma in industrial safety is a one-year full time course with an elaborate syllabus on industrial safety, occupational health and industrial hygiene. This is a qualification that is required to be a safety officer in industries, ports and construction works as per the statutes. There are some compulsory and optional subjects in this course. One compulsory subject contains the syllabus on occupational health, industrial hygiene and personal protective equipment.

This book covers almost all aspects of the syllabus of PDIS/ADIS course. It also contains a 'Miscellaneous' chapter which may be very much related to some of the other subjects of the course. It also contains a chapter called "Notifiable Occupational Diseases: Pictographs" that is required for practical presentation of the subject.

I hope the book will help the students of postgraduate course on industrial safety as well as the safety, health, hygiene, management of industrial as well as corporate personnel to know that health and environment is the essential component of safety in industry.

SK Haldar

Contents

Syllabus

Occupational Health

Meaning of occupational health and occupational health hazards. Awareness programme, types of occupational health hazards—physical, chemical, biological, mechanical and psychosocial hazards. Common work related or occupational diseases—occupations involving risk of contracting those diseases—mode of causation of diseases and its effects—diagnostic methods—methods of prevention—notifiable occupational diseases—compensation of occupational diseases—evaluation of injuries—medical service in industrial establishment and its functions—occupational health service and its activity—occupational hazards in hospital—action programme for work related diseases at the national level—major accident hazards control—medical provision—occupational health audit and survey. Occupational diseases relating to construction work, emergency medical treatment of injuries and rehabilitation at construction site.

Industrial Hygiene

Concept, definition and importance of hygiene in industry. Difference between domestic hygiene and industrial hygiene. Physical hazards—heat stress and its control, ventilation, noise, vibration, improper illumination, thermal radiation—X-ray—ultraviolet radiation—ionizing and non-ionizing radiations—permissible industrial exposure limits—effects of exposure—preventive and control measures.

Noise and vibration—the effect of noise on man, measurement and evaluation of noise, vibration damping, noise isolation, noise absorption—silencers, practical aspect of control of noise. Case studies on impact of noise from compressors and generators. Vibration: effect, measurement and control.

Industrial Physiology

Classification of workload—work capacity and man-job alignment—fatigue and rest allowances—physiological test in occupational health assessment—ergonomics—man-machine differences—man-machine interface—fitting the man to the job—prevention of work-related limb disorders and repetitive strain injury (RSI).

Personal Protective Equipment

Introduction and requirements of PPE. Type of PPE:

a. Non-respiratory personal protective devices: Head protection—ear protection—face and eye protection—head protection—feet protection—body protection—supply. Use, care and maintenance of personal protective equipment—requirement under Factories Act and Rules.
b. Respiratory personal protective devices: Classification of hazards—classification of respiratory personal protective devices—selection of respirators—inspection and hints in the use of breathing apparatus—supply. Use, care and maintenance of breathing apparatus—training in the use of breathing apparatus.

Chapter

1

Occupational Health

MEANING OF OCCUPATIONAL HEALTH AND OCCUPATIONAL HEALTH HAZARD

Occupational Health

Occupational health is the promotion and maintenance of the highest degree of physical, mental and social well-being of the workers in all occupations. It should aim at the promotion and maintenance of the highest degree of physical, mental and social well-being of workers in all occupations, the prevention among workers of departure from health caused by their working conditions; the protection of workers in their employment from risks resulting from factors adverse to health; the placing and maintenance of the worker in an environment adapted to his physiological and psychological capabilities and, to summarize, the adaptation of work to man and of each man to his work. It is a division of general medicine which is devoted to the prevention of occupational disease and injury and to the promotion of health of people at work.

Today's concept of occupational health has greatly been changed from yesterday's concept of 'industrial health'. Now, it is changing to 'environmental health' because of greater awareness of all concerned about the ecological problems arising from rapid industrialization, urbanization, use of complex process and hazardous chemicals in industries.

The modern industrial processes present many hazards to the health of the employees. It is an established fact that there is no occupation which does not have any hazard. It is also true that there is no effective way of cure available for many of the occupational diseases. But there is a rosy part also that most of the occupational diseases are preventable. Preventive medicine and occupational health have the same aim. One of the declared aims of occupational health is to provide a safe occupational environment in order to safeguard the health of the workers and to step up industrial production and development.

Hazard and Risk

Hazard is the potential for causing harm and risk is the likelihood (or, the probability) that such harm will result. The term risk is now extended to include consideration of the severity of effect. If handling sheets of paper at work is just as likely to cause cuts (paper cut) to the skin, as sharpening knives, the probability of injury from both processes is the same, but cut from knives are more severe than paper cuts. Therefore, of the two processes with equal likelihood of skin injury, sharpening knives is viewed as riskier because of the severity of the effect. The distinction between hazard and risk is important in regard to choose to suitable measures to reduce the likelihood of occupational injury or disease. Minimizing risk may be more cost-effective than eliminating hazards.

Occupational environment is the sum of external conditions and influences prevailed at the place of work and which have direct and/or indirect effects on the health of working populations. If occupational environment is polluted, it will affect the health of working population and may cause occupational disease or hazard. The disease which arises out of or in course of occupation is known as *occupational disease* (Fig. 1.1).

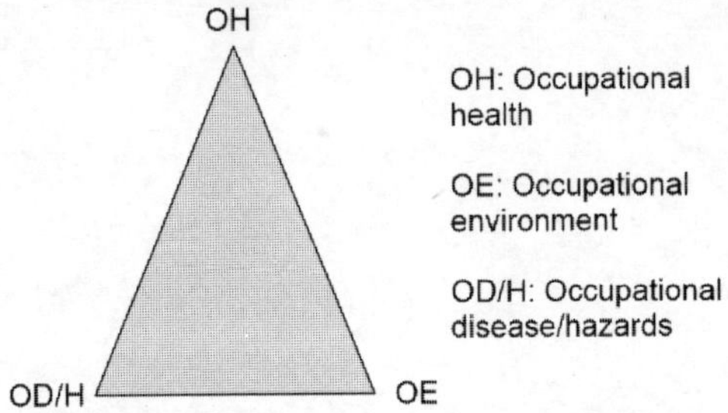

Fig. 1.1: Trangle of interrelation between OH, OE and OD/H

Improvement of environmental health is a major concern of many industries. The objective of health education in environmental health promotion through improvement of personal hygiene are to:

1. Educate the people in the principle of environmental health with a view to bring about desired changes in health practice.
2. Secure adoption, wide use and maintenance of environmental health practice.
3. Promote active participation of the people to improve the personal and environmental health.

An agent is defined as a substance living or non-living or a force, tangible or intangible the excessive presence or relative lack of which may initiate or perpetuate a disease process. Basically, there are three types of interactions in a working environment between environment and hazardous agents, they are:

1. Workers vs physical, chemical and biological agents.
2. Workers vs machine, tools, housekeeping.
3. Workers vs workers.

OCCUPATIONAL HEALTH HAZARDS

An industrial worker may be exposed to five types of hazards, depending upon his occupation:

1. *Physical hazard*: Physical hazard is due to the interaction between workers and physical agents. Examples of physical agents are heat, cold, noise, vibration, ionizing radiation, non-ionizing radiation, illumination, barometric pressure, electricity, electromagnetic fields (EMF).
2. *Chemical hazard*: Chemical hazard is due to the interaction between workers and chemical agents (Fig. 1.2). Chemical hazards are due to excessive airborne concentrations of vapors, gases, or aerosols in the form of dusts, fumes, or mists. These may present an inhalation hazard; some may act as skin irritants or be toxic by absorption through the skin and gastrointestinal tract.

   There is hardly any industry which does not make use of chemicals. The ill effects produced depend upon:

   a. Nature of exposure
   b. Severity of exposure

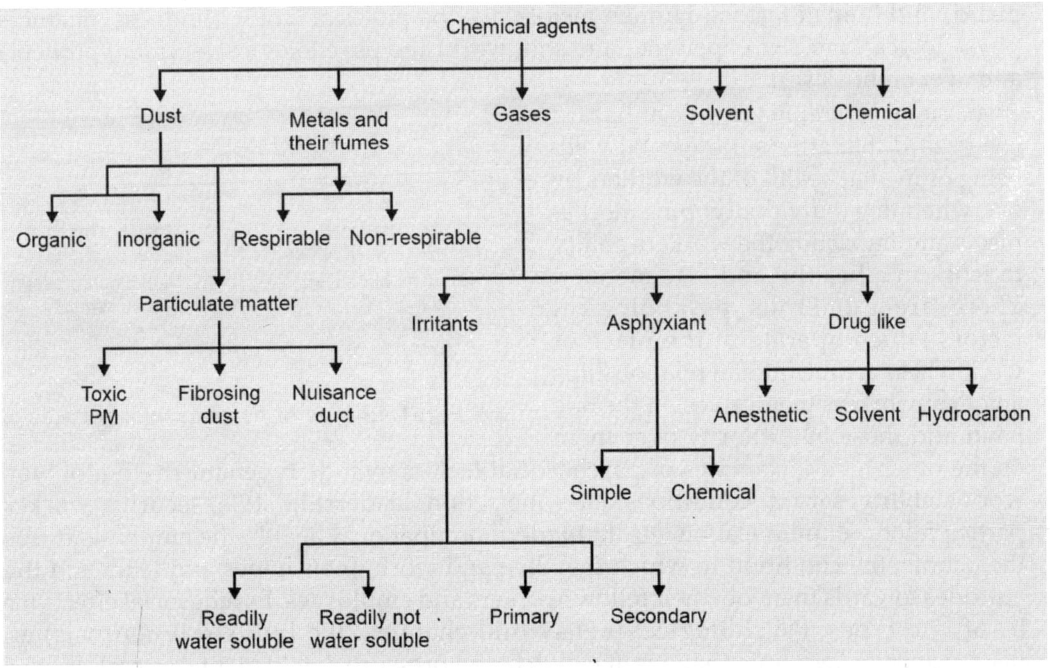

Fig. 1.2: Type of chemical agents

  c. Duration of exposure
  d. Quantum of exposure
  e. Individual susceptibility

3. *Biological hazard*: Biological hazard is due to the interaction between workers and biological agents. Examples are bacteria, virus, and fungus, insects, etc. These hazards may be produced by handling or processing biological specimens, plants, or animals and by improper removal of waste or sewage; inadequate food handling procedures; and deficiencies in personal hygiene, sanitation, and housekeeping procedures. Occupational biohazards may act as infectious, allergenic, toxic, or carcinogenic agents in humans.
4. *Mechanical hazard*: Mechanical hazard is due to the interaction between workers and machine, tools, housekeeping, etc. The unguarded machine, protruding and moving parts, poor installation of the plant, lack of safety measures are the causes of accidents which is a major problem in industries (Fig. 1.3). Working for long hours in un-physiological postures is the cause of fatigue, backache, diseases of joints and muscles and impairment of the workers' health and efficiency. Accident, injuries and cumulative trauma disorder are the examples of mechanical hazards. Factors responsible for mechanical hazard are two: environmental factors (heat, noise, vibration and machine without any

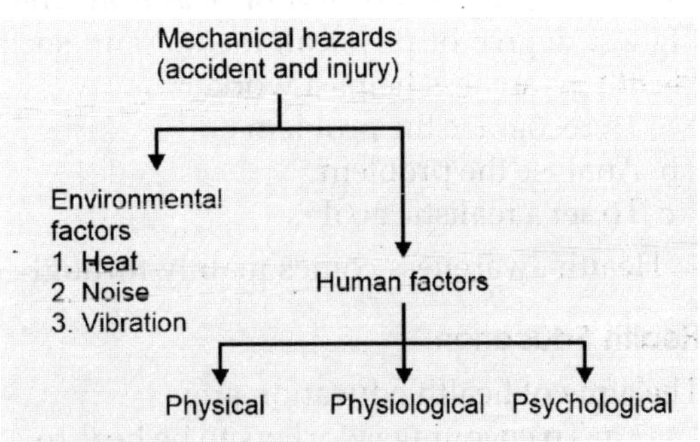

Fig. 1.3: Factors responsible for mechanical hazards

guard) and human factors. Human factors may be physical (color blindness, deafness), physiological (age, sex, experience and shift work) and psychological (accident proneness and over enthusiasm).

5. *Psychosocial hazard*: Psychosocial hazard is a hazard that affects the mental well-being or mental health of the workers by overwhelming individual coping mechanisms and impacting the workers ability to work in a healthy and safe manner. There are numerous psychological factors which operate at the place of work. These are the human relationships amongst workers themselves on the one hand and those in authority over them on the other hand. Examples of psychosocial factors include type and rhythm of work, work stability, service conditions, job satisfaction, leadership style, security, workers' participation, communication, etc. In modern occupational health, the emphasis is upon the people, the condition in which they live and work, their hopes and fears and their attitudes towards their job, their fellow-workers and employees. Psychosocial effects may be of two types: Psychological (behavioral changes like industrial neurosis) and psychosomatic (systemic changes like high blood pressure due to mental stress) (Fig. 1.4).

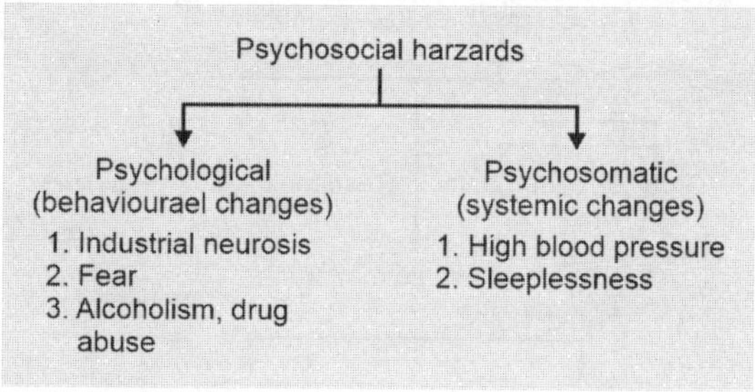

Fig. 1.4: Type of psychosocial hazards

OCCUPATIONAL HEALTH AWARENESS PROGRAMME

There is a growing awareness that improved working conditions and the working environment are a positive contribution to the national development and a necessity in the achievement of sustainable development. But despite the efforts of all concerned, the incidence of diseases is still too high and the workplace remains hazardous. Hazards related to the use of chemicals are widespread and according to ILO estimate, two out of every three workers worldwide are exposed to them. It shows how important it is to multiply our efforts to protect working people and the environment against these hazards. Prevention is the treatment of choice in case of occupational health hazards to save lives of workers and economic losses in industries as well as these are essential for the excellence in industrial development.

Health awareness is a process that bring out changes in workers' knowledge, attitude, skill and behaviour. A positive knowledge, attitude and participation of the employees should be there through the process of health awareness for the promotion and maintenance of the highest degree of physical, mental and social well-being of the workers in all occupations. Health awareness helps a worker:

a. To recognize the problem
b. Analyse the problem
c. To set a realistic goal

Health awareness comes mainly through: (a) Health education; (b) Training.

Health Education

The aims of health education are:

a. To encourage workers to be healthy
b. To know how to stay healthy through scientific information.

The steps of health education are:

a. To culture a health awareness
b. To culture a healthy lifestyle
c. To culture a group responsibility
d. To culture interest, attitude and value.

The practice of health education may be:

a. Individual health education
b. Group health education—through lecture, group discussion, panel discussion, symposium, workshop, role playing, demonstration, programme instruction and simulation exercise.

Training

Workers often experience work related health problems and do not realise that the problems are related to their work, particularly when an occupational disease, e.g. is in the early stage. Besides the other more obvious benefits of training are:

a. Skill development
b. Hazards recognition.

A comprehensive training programme in each workplace will help workers:

a. To recognize early stage/symptom of any potential occupational disease before they become permanent
b. To assess their work environment
c. To insist the management to make changes before hazardous condition can develop. Employee training should be designed to influence employees to comply with appropriate work practice. Such training should be conducted periodically for all employees.

Training should include the following areas:

a. Potential risk of overexposure
b. The importance of industrial hygiene, biological monitoring and notification of test results
c. Description of work practice control including personal protective equipment
d. Firs-aid and emergency training.

WORKPLACE HEALTH PROMOTION

Workplace health promotion is an approach towards health gain by encouragement of all aspects of positive health. It is a process of enabling people to increase their control over their own health and to improve it. It is a continuation towards well-being or optimal health. It also states that health promotion is not just the responsibility of the health sector, and goes beyond healthy lifestyles to well-being. Reduction of health care costs, disability claim and absenteeism and increase in productivity are the benefits of health promotion. Job satisfaction and work stability are also the results of health promotion. Workers' lifestyles may have a specific or a general impact on their health, safety and working capacity. Workers should be advised on avoiding lifestyles harmful to health as well as on adopting healthy and safe working practice.

For occupational health professionals the promotion of health in the workplace means conducting an occupational health practice which involves protecting and promoting workers' health through the prevention of occupational and other work-related injuries and diseases. For specialists in health promotion, it may mean introducing non-smoking policies, tackling alcohol and drug abuse, encouraging physical exercise and healthy diets, changing behavioral patterns, and undertaking activities to bring these things about.

Wellness may be defined as optimal health. Achieving it may involve improving physical and mental ability, developing reserve capacities and adaptability to changing circumstances, and reaching new heights in creative and other work. In a working environment, some of these factors can be evaluated quantitatively in relation to absenteeism, presenteeism, job satisfaction and work stability.

Absenteeism: Absenteeism or absence from work is defined as nonattendance when expected to work, for any reason at all, medical or other. *Presenteeism*: A loss of workplace productivity resulting from employee health problems and/or personal issues even though the employee is physically present at work.

COMMON WORK-RELATED (OCCUPATIONAL) DISEASES OR HAZARDS

Physical Hazards

1. *Heat*: The common physical hazard in most industries is heat. Heat stress is the amount of heat that is to be eliminated from human body to remain the body in thermal equilibrium and estimated as the metabolic heat load and heat loss or gain through the process of convection, conduction, radiation, and evaporation. The direct effects of heat exposure are burn, heat cramps, heat syncope, heat exhaustion, heat hyperpyrexia and heat stroke. The indirect effects of heat are decrease efficiency, increase fatigue, enhanced accident, decrease productivity, sleeplessness and fatigue (Fig. 1.5).

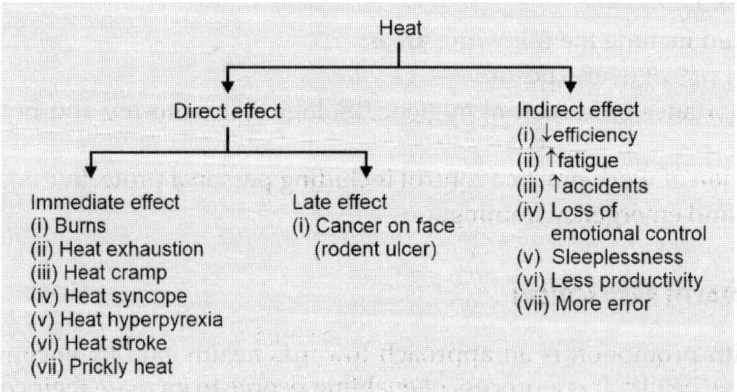

Fig. 1.5: Effect of heat

2. *Cold*: The effect of cold or subnormal atmospheric temperature may be of two types—generalized effect and local effect (Fig. 1.6). Generalized effects include coldness, hypothermia, shivering, weakness, desire to sleep, coma and death. Local effects depend upon the type of subnormal temperature like freezing and non-freezing temperature. Important hazards associated with freezing (ice forming) temperature are frostnip, frostbite (superficial, deep and freeze-thaw-refreeze injury). The example of non-freezing (non-ice forming) temperature is immersion foot or trench foot which is due to the

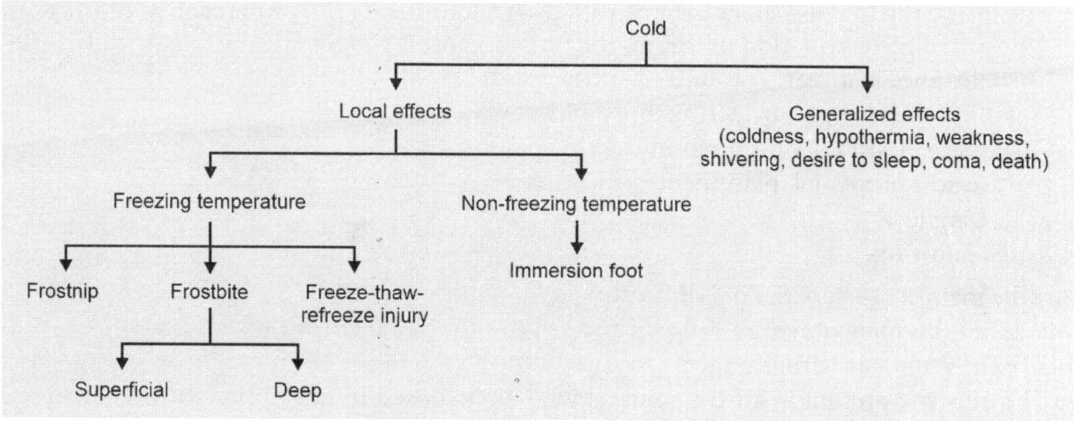

Fig. 1.6: Health effect of cold

immersion of feet in cold water during work usually in standing posture. There may be arterial thrombosis, and sudden cardiac death.

3. *Noise*: According to American National Standard Institute (ANSI), any unwanted sound is known as noise. The characteristics of noise are: Intensity or loudness measured by the unit 'dB' and frequency or sharpness measured by Hz or cycle per second. The effects of noise are two types:
   a. Auditory effect consists of noise induced temporary threshold shift (NITTS) and noise induce hearing loss (NIHL) or noise induced permanent threshold shift (NIPTS)
   b. Non auditory effects.

NITTS: The magnitude of a temporary threshold shift is proportional to the intensity and duration of the stimulus and the recovery. Recovery usually occurs within 16 hours but may take several days with higher intensities. This stage is reversible. The sign of developing permanent threshold shift is a complex process. Interaction between the level, nature and number of noise exposure, their duration and frequency and the individual susceptibility are all factors. Classically, there is high frequency rise in threshold with a characteristic notch at 4 kHz though the notch may center at 3–6 kHz. This is often accompanied by tinnitus and after a short rest period, the rise in threshold recovers. With repeated exposure there is a tendency to acquire resistance to the auditory effects in that the degree of temporary threshold shift lessens though at some arbitrary point continued exposure leads to a permanent threshold shift.

NIPTS/NIHL: When NITTS is repeated for years, it tends to lose the sensitivity to acoustic stimuli due to the destruction of structure in the inner ear (hair cells), thus leading to permanent hearing loss or NIHL. This is characterized by irreversible audiometric effects and pathological changes in the cochlea. The 4 kHz notch tends to deepen in audiogram and also insidiously widen, encompassing adjacent high frequencies. Once the audiometric changes encroach upon the speech frequencies (2–3 kHz in particular) the affected individual becomes aware of the diminished acuity in his or her hearing. Speech discrimination with background noise becomes difficult and the associated tinnitus (which are highly variable in character) may become intrusive. The rate of progression again depends on the noise parameters cited previously and on individual susceptibility. Generally, progression at 4 kHz is initially rapid but slows down after 10–12 years. The deafness due to noise in industry is called sensory neural (SN) or perceptive deafness. In the hearing conservation program, the noise-exposed people are audiometrically tested usually once in a year. The aims of such periodic examination are to:

a. Observe changes in hearing threshold.
b. Assess the ability to communicate.
c. Assess proper job placement.
d. Diagnose
e. Follow up.

The main characteristics of NIHL are:

a. It is permanent
b. It is subtle in earlier stage
c. It is not present in all the subjects who are exposed to noise. Hence, protection and periodic audiometric examination for all the noised exposed people are essential.

Non-auditory effect of noise:

a. It is a common observation that any sudden noise will produce 'startle' reaction in anyone and it cannot be voluntarily controlled. It can occur even during sleep. The characteristics of startle reaction are:
    i. The blood vessels contract
    ii. Blood pressure increases
    iii. Pupil dilates
    iv. Both voluntary and involuntary muscles become tense (contract). After a few minutes startle reaction becomes normal.
b. Noise stimulates adrenal glands to produce hormone catecholamines and this hormone is responsible for certain heart and circulatory diseases.
c. Nausea and vomiting.
d. Pulse and respiratory rates increase.
e. Noise increases physical and psychological stresses.
f. Sleeplessness
g. Fatigue.
h. Irritability and socially undesirable behavior.
i. It reduces work efficiency and productivity.
j. Increases accident and error.
k. Tiredness and insomnia.
l. Peptic ulcer.
m. Sickness absenteeism and presenteeism.
n. Tendency to speak loudly.

4. *Vibration*: Vibration are two types: Hand-arm vibration (HAV) and whole-body vibration (WBV). The unit of vibration is Hz or cycle per second. Occupational vibration reaches the worker through different paths or transmission routes (Fig. 1.7). In 'whole-body vibration' it is conducted through a contacting or supporting structure that is itself vibrating, like a ship's deck, the seat of a vehicle traversing rough terrain, a vibrating platform. In other industrial processes, the route of entry is through paths to the hands, wrists and arms of the subjects, so-called 'segmental vibration' or 'hand-arm vibration'. The examples of tools producing hand-arm vibration are pneumatic tools, electric-driven grinding, burrowing

tools, rock drilling, and cross cutting timber. The prolonged use of vibrating tools and equipment can lead to a number of pathological effects. Hand-arm vibration may cause hand-arm vibration syndrome (HAVS) like white finger and whole-body vibration may cause motion sickness and low back pain.

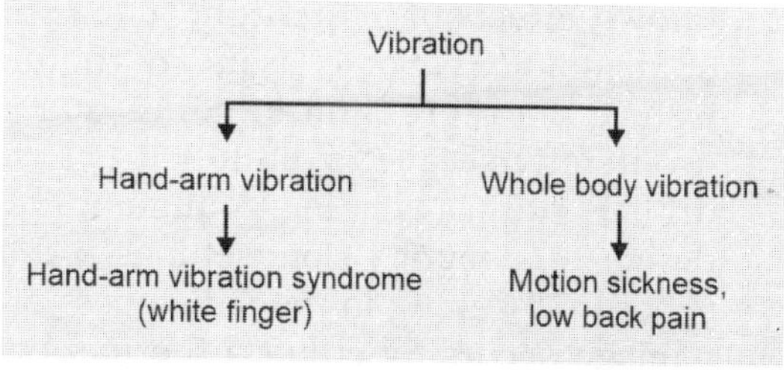

Fig. 1.7: Health hazard of vibration

5. *Non-ionizing radiation*: The electromagnetic radiation spectrum has been divided into a number of frequency regions. The most useful divisions are between ionizing (X-rays, gamma rays, cosmic rays) and non-ionizing radiation (ultraviolet radiation, visible rays, infrared radiation, radiofrequency waves) (Fig. 1.8). Non-ionizing radiation is that part of the electromagnetic spectrum which does not have sufficient energy to ionize matter, but can excite atoms by raising their outer electrons to higher orbitals, a process which may store energy, produce heat or cause chemical reaction (photochemistry).

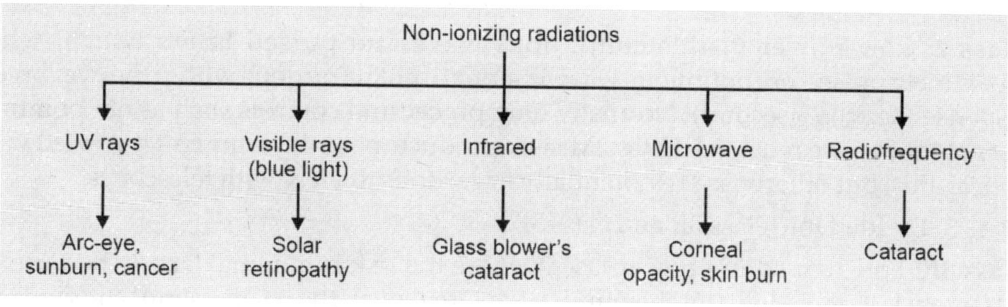

Fig. 1.8: Health hazard of non-ionizing radiations

Ultraviolet radiation (UV ray) may produce 'arc eye' or 'flash eye' and skin burn. Sources of UV radiation such as welding arcs must be shielded from workers near the operation with use of materials opaque to UV to prevent 'arc eye' or 'flash eye'. Excessive exposure of the eyes to *infrared (IR)* from furnaces and other hot bodies has traditionally been thought to produce 'glass blower's cataract' or 'heat cataract'. Overexposure to near infrared may also damage the retina by protein denaturation. Chronic exposure to excessive IR can also cause a 'dry eye' irritation of cornea. Acute, accidental exposure of the eyes to microwave radiation may lead to skin burns, conjunctival infection and loss of corneal epithelium, as well as stromal edema and opacification. Long-term exposure of radiofrequency may produce some adverse effects include nervous, neuroendocrine, reproductive, immune and sensory system effects, cataracts formation, decrease birthweight, behavioral changes.

LASER: Laser is an acronym for light amplification by the stimulated emission of radiation. Lasers are sources of non-ionizing radiation that can operate in the UV, visible and infrared region of the electromagnetic spectrum. The light emitted has a unique combination of spatial coherence (all the waves are in step), monochromaticity (one color or narrow wavelength range) and usually high collimation. Furthermore, the emission may be continuous wave or pulsed for either long or short (Q-switched) duration. The known effects of acute light damage to ocular tissues are exploited in preventive ophthalmology. Some lasers are routinely used in retinal scatter photocoagulation to induce the regression of subretinal and preretinal vessels in conditions such as proliferative diabetic retinopathy. Lasers are commonly used both in industry (e.g. drilling, cutting, welding, communication) and military (e.g. rangefinders, tactical target designators, night vision) settings and there have been numerous reports of accidental exposure resulting in immediate loss of central vision. Depending on the type of laser, damage occurs by either a thermal or mechanical mechanism. It may cause retinal damage. In addition to potential optic hazards, lasers may create airborne contaminants generated by the process or the laser fuels used, including noise, fire, electrical, and cryogenic hazards. A laser impacting on a hazardous metal part, e.g. could generate a fume and other small particles.

Classifications of laser are defined by the American National Standards Institute (ANSI) Z-136.1: 2007 and British Standard BS/EN/IEC 6082:2007:

Class 1: Non-hazardous lasers:

i. The output is so low the laser is inherently safe
ii. The laser is part of a totally enclosed system. A class 1M laser product is safe to view without optical aids, but otherwise is potentially hazardous.

Class 2: Low power visible continuous wave and pulsed lasers which, whether repetitively pulsed or continuous wave lasers, are not hazardous within the eye's aversion response (i.e. $\leq$0.25 second). Normally only procedural controls such as not pointing the laser at the eye are required. Class 2M laser products pose the same risk if viewed without optical aids, but otherwise are potentially hazardous to view with telescopes.

Class 3: Divided into class 3R and class 3B.

Class 3R: Low to medium power lasers where the risk is minimal largely because of the extremely low probability of the pupil being large, of all the beam energy entering the eye and the eye accommodated to focus the beam to a minimal spot. Nevertheless, the eye may be exposed technically to levels up to five times the maximum possible exposure (MPE). Hazard can be controlled by relatively simple procedures (e.g. use of beam stops and ensuring that beam paths are not at eye level). The only documented injuries from this type of laser have occurred from intentional direct-beam exposure.

Class 3B: Medium power lasers where the viewing beam either directly or by specular reflection is hazardous, but diffuse reflections are almost always safe. Hazard can be controlled by the use of beam enclosure, beam stops (ensuring that beam paths are not at eye level) and, it needed laser eye protection.

Class 4: High power lasers which are not only a hazard from direct viewing and from specular reflections, but also from diffuse reflections. The direct beam may also be a skin and fire hazard. Their use requires extreme caution.

6. *Ionizing radiation*: The radiation which can penetrate the human cells and deposits its energy within it is known as ionizing radiation (Fig. 1.9). The effects of ionizing radiation are:
   a. Somatic effects consist of:
      i. Immediate effects like ionizing burn, radiation sickness and acute radiation syndrome
      ii. Delayed effect like leukemia, carcinogenesis, fetal developmental abnormalities and shortening of life.

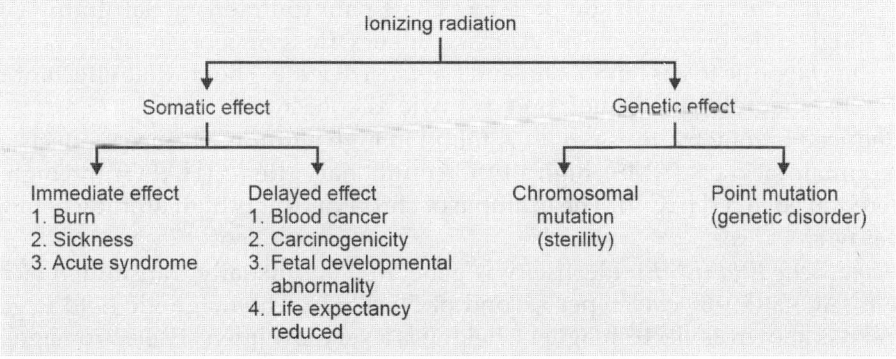

Fig. 1.9: Health effect of ionizing radiation

b. Genetic effects these are:
   i. Chromosomal mutation—causes sterility
   ii. Point mutation—affects gene.

7. *Illumination*: The workers may be exposed to the risk of poor illumination or excessive brightness. The acute effects of poor illumination are eye strain, headache, eye pain, lacrimation, congestion around the cornea, eye fatigue, etc. The chronic effect of poor illumination is 'miner's nystagmus'. Exposure to excessive brightness or 'glare' is associated with discomfort, annoyance and visual fatigue. Intense direct glare may also result in blurring of vision and lead to accident.
8. *Atmospheric pressure*: Atmospheric or environmental pressure may be high or low (Fig. 1.10).
   a. High barometric pressure: The increases of barometric pressure which have been experienced by the sea depth as great as 701 m (7000 kPa), some 70 times the normal barometric pressure present at the earth's surface (100 kPa). Acute effects may be two types:
      i. Compression barotrauma: Effects during work at high atmospheric pressure within the caisson or working at the bottom of sea or tunnelling work are middle and inner ear barotrauma, sinus pain, teethache, etc.
      ii. Decompression illness: Health effects occur when coming back to normal atmosphere from high barometric pressure. The effects are musculoskeletal pain,

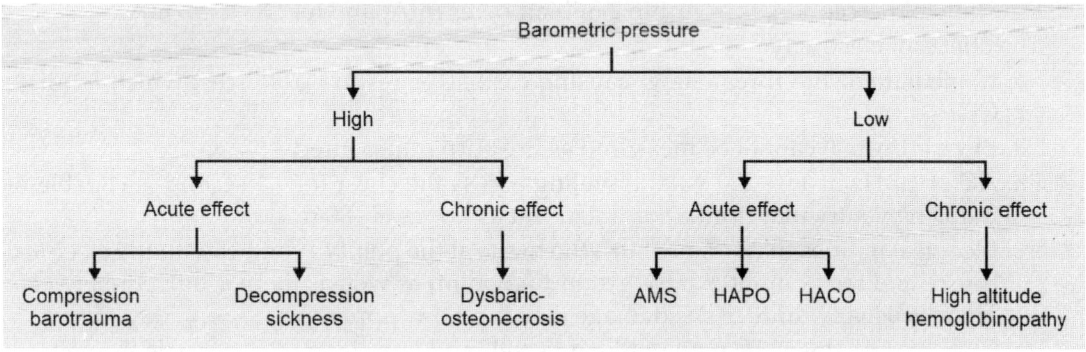

Fig. 1.10: Health hazard of barometric pressure

cardiopulmonary decompression, chest pain (pulmonary barotraumas), neurological decompression (psychosis), latency (loss of consciousness on coming to surface due to gas embolism) and Caison's disease. The chronic effects are hearing loss, neurological sequela and dysbaric osteonecrosis.

b. Reduced barometric pressure: It is found in high altitude. The acute effects are acute mountain sickness (AMS), high altitude pulmonary edema (HAPO) and high-altitude cerebral edema (HACO). The example of chronic effect is high altitude hemoglobinopathy.

9. *Electromagnetic field (EMF)*: Electricity is generated and usually transmitted as alternate current (AC) at 50–60 cycles per second or 50–60 Hz. The magnetic field is generated around it is known as electromagnetic field. It is a very low intensity electromagnetic field. Electromagnetic field (EMF) is measured in tesla (T) or micro-tesla (mT), are determined by the ACGIH's ceiling value (at 60 Hz magnetic field) for guideline exposure limit is 1 mT. EMF is available around every electrical conductor, motor, electrical appliances, House wiring, current floor on the safety grounding system, utility line outside the home, computers, copy machine, power distribution facility and large motor, near large electric machine, electrical heating equipment, television, cellular phone and radar. Long-term health effects are:
   a. Cancer formation: Leukemia (blood cancer), brain cancer, breast cancer, lung cancer, malignant melanoma, cancer of prostate, testes and pituitary gland.
   b. Reproductive effects are:
      i. Parental exposure and brain tumor: If father is exposed then offspring may develop childhood brain tumor, neuroblastoma.
      ii. Pregnancy outcomes: Spontaneous abortion and congenital malformation.
   c. Neurobehavioral and neurogenerative effects: General neurasthenic effects—depressive symptoms, suicidal tendency, Alzheimer's disease. EMF has definite effect on pacemaker.

10. *Electricity*: The nature and severity of electrical injury depend on:
   a. The type and voltage of electrical current.
   b. The resistance of the body at the point of entry of electrical current.
   c. The pathway of the current flowing through the body.
   d. The duration of exposure.

   Alternate current (AC) produces greater damage than a direct current (DC) of the same amperage. The AC flow of 60 cycles (Hz) that will produce a tingling sensation, the threshold of perception, is from 1 to 2 milliamperes (mA) and for DC it is 5 mA.

   The effects of electricity:
   i. Immediate or life-threatening, causing cardiac or respiratory arrest which requires CPR.
   ii. Electric burn. It cannot be measured as fire burn is measured.
   iii. AC of 60 Hz at 110–220 volts traveling across the chest for <1 second is capable of inducing ventricular fibrillation at current as low as 60–80 mA.
   iv. Electrical injuries may visibly burn the tissue at the point of contact with the electrical source and the point of exit (or grounding point) as well as there is burn in-between. There is usually more tissue damage than is readily apparent.
   v. Current flow flows the path of blood vessels and muscles and may cause thrombosis and necrosis of tissue at sites remote from the apparent injury.

vi. There may be associated musculoskeletal injuries not only from the titanic contraction of muscles but also from the not uncommon fall of the electrically injured victim.
vii. Oliguria due to renal damage may be a sequela of electrical injury due to destruction of muscles and the production of myoglobin pigment in the urine.
viii. Severe pain.
ix. Dehydration.
x. Shock and death.

Chemical Hazards

Hazards due to gases:

1. *Carbon monoxide (CO) poisoning*: CO poisoning is the most common of all poisoning in industry today. It is known as 'silent killer' because it is colorless, odorless, tasteless and non-irritant, therefore, gives no warming of its presence under any circumstances. It is a chemical asphyxiant. The mechanisms of toxicity are:
   a. It has 200–300 times more affinity towards hemoglobin than oxygen and produces carboxyhemoglobin. Therefore, cells will not get oxygen for cellular respiration.
   b. It inhibits cytochrome A_3 oxidase (cytochrome-monoxide binding) at the cellular level.

   The acute effects are dizziness, nausea, weakness and collapse. Acute heavy exposure may result in loss of consciousness without warning, followed by coma, convulsion and death. The classical cherry pink color of the skin is a rare sign but venous blood frequently looks arterial. Patient recovering from CO poisoning may suffer neurological sequelae including tremor, personality changes, memory impairment, loss of visual acuity, inability to concentrate and parkinsonian features. Moist oxygen inhalation or in some cases hyperbaric oxygen therapy is the treatment of choice.
2. *Hydrogen cyanide (HCN) poisoning*: Hydrogen cyanide is a chemical asphyxiant. Hydrogen cyanide and its sodium, potassium and calcium salts manifest their toxicity by way of a common mechanism, namely, inhibition of the respiratory enzyme cytochrome oxidase. The inhibition causes cellular anoxia and, if a large enough dose is received, results in death. Victims of acute poisoning present with headache, dizziness and vertigo. There may be agitation and confusion, with nausea and vomiting. Acute cyanide poisoning induces sustained seizures, endogenous catecholamine release and cardiovascular shock. Skin contact with solution of cyanide salt can cause itching, discoloration or corrosion. Cyanide salt aerosols can cause upper respiratory irritation. Enlargement of the thyroid gland has also been reported. An increased occurrence of the objective symptoms of headache, changes in taste and smell, irritation of the throat, vomiting, breathlessness on effort, lacrimation, abdominal colic, precordial pain and nervous instability has been noted among workers having long-term occupational exposure to low concentration of HCN.
3. *Hydrogen sulfide*: Hydrogen sulfide is acute acting toxic substance and a leading cause of sudden death in the workplace. It is a chemical asphyxiant. Brief exposure at high concentrations cause unconsciousness, respiratory paralysis and death. Eye irritation, cough, sore throat, vague gastrointestinal symptoms and photophobia may occur with low-level exposure, with overwhelming exposure, collapse and respiratory arrest can develop within minutes.
4. *Ammonia*: Ammonia is a colorless gas and is one of the most widely used industrial chemicals ranking forth in volume of production after sulfuric acid, lime and oxygen.

Ammonia vapor is a severe irritant to the eyes, respiratory tract and skin. It may cause corneal irritation, breathlessness, bronchospasm, chest pain and pulmonary edema that may be fatal. Production of pink frothy sputum often occurs. Complication can include bronchitis or pneumonia. Liquid anhydrous ammonia in contact with the eyes may cause serious eye injury or blindness, on the skin, it causes first and second-degree burns that often are severe and if extensive, may be fatal.

5. *Chlorine*: Chlorine gas is a severe irritant of the eyes, mucous membrane, skin and respiratory system. A major accidental exposure to unmeasured but high concentration for a brief period caused burning of the eyes with lacrimation, burning of nose and mouth with rhinorrhea, cough, choking sensation and substernal pain. These symptoms frequently were accompanied by nausea, vomiting, headache, dizziness and sometime syncope.
6. *Sulfur dioxide*: It is a severe irritant for the eyes, mucous membrane and skin. Exposure to concentration 10 to 50 ppm for 5 to 15 minutes causes irritation of eyes, nose and throat, rhinorrhoea, choking, cough, reflex bronchoconstriction. The liquid form may cause corneal and skin burns.
7. *Benzene:* Inhalation of high concentration of benzene (3000–7500 ppm) may cause a state of excitation and euphoria (benzol jag) followed by drowsiness, fatigue, vertigo, nausea and vomiting, convulsion followed by paralysis, loss of consciousness and death from respiratory failure. Inhalation of small amount of benzene over a long period has caused blood dyscrasias, including aplastic anemia, leukemia (blood cancer), thrombocytopenia. Additional signs and symptoms of chronic toxicity may include headache, dizziness, fatigue, loss of appetite, irritability, nervousness, nose bleeding and other hemorrhagic manifestation.
8. *Phosgene*: In most fatal cases, pulmonary edema reaches a maximum in 12 hours followed by death in 24–48 hours. With moderate exposure the presenting symptoms often are a dryness or a burning sensation in the throat, vomiting, pain in the chest, and dyspnea. Delayed onset of pulmonary edema is characterized by cough, abundant 'foamy' sputum, progressive dyspnea, and severe cyanosis. Pulmonary edema may progress to pneumonia, and cardiac failure may intervene. Exposure to high concentrations may also cause severe conjunctivitis and subsequent turbidity of the cornea of eye. Chronic bronchitis and emphysema have been reported as a consequence of acute exposure. Because of the often-delayed onset of symptom following potentially lethal exposures of phosgene, education of employees and medical observation following suspected overexposure are extremely important. Medical examinations, including pulmonary function tests, are necessary to evaluate recovery from overexposure and to detect chronic lung changes.
9. *Methyl isocyanate*: It is a widely used chemical, but it gained worldwide notoriety after its disastrous release from the Union Carbide pesticide plant in Bhopal, India in 1984. It was being used in the chemical synthesis of carbaryl pesticides, and had been stored in liquid form in two steel tanks. The cause of the incident is still not known, but at 00.30 on December 3, 1984 an exothermic reaction took place in one of the storage tanks, resulting in the escape over a few hours of 40 tons of methyl isocyanate. A dense cloud of methyl isocyanate flowed over an area of the city about 40 km^2 at a time when there was a temperature inversion and a light wind. It is considered that >10000 people were killed and hundreds of thousands injured in the disaster. Methyl isocyanate is an intense

lacrimator and irritates eyes, mucous membrane and skin. The liquid in contact with the eye may cause permanent damage. It may cause pulmonary irritation and sensitization. Exposure of man to high concentration can cause cough, dyspnea, increase secretions and chest pain.

10. *Carbon dioxide*: It is a colorless and odorless gas but when breathed from an anesthetic machine it has a faintly acid smell. The effects of breathing carbon dioxide are very characteristic. 2–3% CO_2 in air will pass unnoticed at rest, but tidal volume is increased by 30% and the minute volume by 5%; on exertion there may be marked shortness of breath. At 3% CO_2 in air, breathing becomes noticeably deeper and more frequent at rest, with the effect becoming more marked until at 5% CO_2 in air there is severe dyspnea, with limits exposure for most people. Subjects complain of headache and are sweaty and have a bounding pulse. At 10% CO_2 in air, respiratory distress develops rapidly with loss of consciousness in 10–15 minutes, even though the oxygen concentration is reduced to 19% only. Exposure to carbon dioxide levels above 15% are intolerable and rapid loss of consciousness ensues after a few breaths of a mixture of 30% carbon dioxide in air. Even at this level, the oxygen concentration is 15%, not enough to cause loss of consciousness from hypoxia, but death will occur if the carbon dioxide level is maintained. Thus, it is important to note that monitoring oxygen in air is an inadequate guide to the carbon dioxide hazard; carbon dioxide should be directly measured. A working or living area should be immediately evacuated when concentration exceed 1.5% by volume (the occupational short-term exposure limit value). Carbon dioxide absorbs the solar energy and prevents the energy from radiating back into the space. As a result, the atmosphere gets heated up. This is commonly known as the greenhouse effect that causes global warming. Normally, the heat from the sun is radiated to the earth and this heat is again radiated back into the space.

Hazards due to Dusts

The term 'pneumoconiosis' is defined by the Fourth International Conference of experts in 1971 as 'the accumulation of dust in the lungs and the tissue reaction to its presence'.

Diseases	*Causes*	*Source of dust*
1. Baritosis	Barium sulfate	Mines of barium sulfate
2. Siderosis	Iron oxide	Welding
3. Stannosis	Tin oxide	Smelting
4. Kaolinosis	Hydrated aluminum silicate	China clay
5. Aluminosis	Stamped aluminum	Paints
6. Anthracosis/CWP	Coal dust	Coal mining
7. Silicosis	Free silica dust	Mining, quarrying, etc.
8. Talcosis	Hydrated magnesium silicate	Rubber industry
9. Berylliosis	Beryllium compounds	Atomic reactor, aero engineering
10. Asbestosis	Asbestos fiber	Mining, brake lining, asbestos-cement product

Damage to the lungs caused by dust or fumes or noxious substances inhaled by workers in certain specific occupations is known as *occupational lung disease (OLD)*. All pneumoconiosis(s) are OLD but all OLD are not pneumoconiosis. Pneumoconiosis is defined as "the accumulation

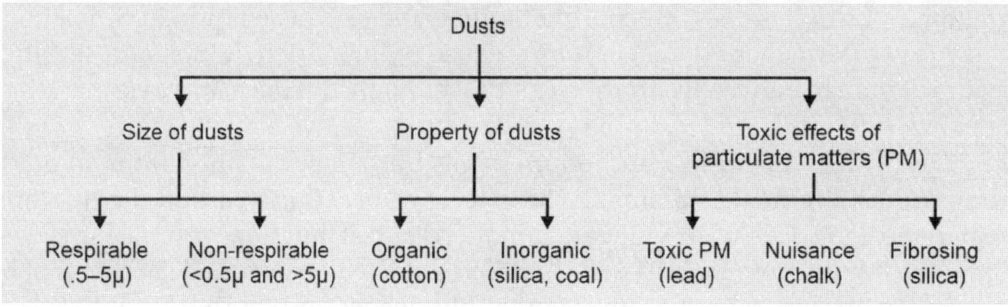

Fig. 1.11: Types of dusts

of dust in the lungs and the tissue reactions to its presence". The clinical and pathological consequences that result from the inhalation of dust are variable mainly according to (Fig. 1.11):

1. The properties of the dust
2. The intensity and the duration of the exposure
3. Host susceptibility.

Dust constitutes one of the most common respiratory hazards. Dusts may be *respirable* (0.5–5 microns in diameter) or *non-respirable* (below 0.5 micron and above 5 micron), or dusts may be *organic* like cotton, tobacco or sugar cain fibre, or *inorganic/mineral dusts* like silica, coal dust, asbestos, or, dusts may be:

1. *Toxic particulate matter:* When these dusts are inhaled, they will not be restricted/retained in the lungs but they will be absorbed in the system for toxic systemic effects, e.g. lead, cadmium, chromium dusts.
2. *Fibrosing dusts*: When these dusts are inhaled, they will be retained in the lungs and produce fibrosis of the lung tissue, e.g. free silica, coal dusts and asbestos fiber.
3. *Nuisance dusts*: In contrast to fibrogenic dusts which cause scar tissue in lungs when inhaled in excess amounts, so-called 'nuisance' dust has a long history little adverse effect on lungs and do not produce significant organic disease or toxic effect when exposures are kept under reasonable control. The nuisance dusts have also been called (biologically) 'inert' dusts, but the later term is inappropriate to the extent that there is no dust which does not evoke some cellular response in the lung when inhaled in sufficient amount. Example of nuisance dust is chalk dust.

Some Common Pneumoconiosis

1. *Silicosis*: Silicosis is a fibrotic disease of the lung caused by the inhalation of, retention of and pulmonary reaction to crystalline silica. The three important crystalline form of silica are quartz, tridymite, and cristobalite. These forms are also called free silica to distinguish them from the silicates. There is mounting evidence that freshly fractured silica may be more toxic than aged silica, perhaps related to reactive radical groups on the cleavage planes of freshly fractured silica. This may offer a pathogenic explanation for the observation of cases of advanced disease in both sandblasters and rock drillers where exposure to recently fractured silica is particularly intense.

   Types of silicosis: Acute silicosis, chronic silicosis and accelerated silicosis.

   Complications of Silicosis:

   a. Tuberculosis and other infection: When active tuberculosis is common in the community, many patients with silicosis develop combined diseases with an extremely poor prognosis and called 'silicotuberculosis'.

b. Progressive massive fibrosis (PMF).
c. Pulmonary heart disease (cor pulmonale).
d. Rheumatoid syndrome: With high titers of circulating rheumatoid factor without overt arthropathy.
e. Nephropathy: Kidney damage with proteinuria and systemic hypertension.
f. Carcinogenicity: It can produce cancer.

Prevention: There is no specific therapy for silicosis. Prevention remains the cornerstone of eliminating this occupational lung disease. Prevention of silicosis depends on preventing exposure to respiratory silica dust which presupposes that the risk has been recognized; regrettably this is not always the case. Most countries now recognize a silica dust standard aimed at preventing exposure of the workforce to more than permissible level of quartz. Ideally, the use of quart should be avoided if a safer substitute material is available. There is some evidence that inhalation of quartz mixed with other dusts leads to a less severe and progressive disease. The education of workers and employers regarding the hazards of silica dust exposure and measures to control exposure is important. Improved ventilation and local exhaust, process enclosure, wet technique, personal protection including the proper selection of respirators and where possible, industrial substitution of agents less hazardous than silica reduces exposure. Silicosis is a reportable disease. Workers exposed to a risk of silicosis should be offered chest radiography at regular intervals, probably at least once in every 3 years, in order that the earliest signs of disease are detected and the workers protected from further exposure. If silicosis is recognized in a worker, limited future significant exposure is advisable. Unfortunately, the disease may progress even without further silica exposure.

2. *Asbestosis and asbestos fiber*: The mineral known as asbestos, a name derived from the Greek word for unquenchable, belongs to one of two mineralogical groups, the serpentines and amphiboles. Asbestos is a collective term for some of the metamorphic, fibrous, mineral silicate. Chrysotile or white asbestos is the only asbestos that is a serpentine; it is a magnesium silicate with a curly configuration and is able to shear into many smaller fibrils. It is a soft and silky fiber, has high tensile strength, high flexibility, good spin ability and high resistance to alkali. It undergoes thermal decomposition at about 675°C. All the other forms of asbestos are amphiboles. This group of minerals consists of a large number of structurally similar but chemically different chemicals. It is straight and needle like fiber. It is generally more brittle and appears to be dustier. It has greater resistance to acid and heat. Asbestos has a long history. It was first used in Finland about 2500 BC to strengthen clay pot. In Greek it was used as 'magic cloth' which did not burn in fire. Asbestos is derived from the Greek word meaning 'inextinguishable' or 'indestructible'. They have different physical and chemical properties, but share a fibrous form or habit. Mineralogists have generally taken a particle with a length-to-breath ratio (aspect ratio) of 10 : 1 or more to be a fiber (as per the Indian Factories Act, 1948, TLV of asbestos fiber is for fiber >5 μm in length and <5 μm in breath with length to breath ratio equal to or >3 : 1). Prevention and screening of asbestos related hazards are: Screening of asbestos-exposed populations can be carried out for practical and scientific purposes. There are four goals of screening: to identify high-risk groups, to target preventive actions, to discover occupational diseases, to develop improved tools for treatment, rehabilitation and prevention. Of the three routes of exposure (dermal, ingestion and inhalation) to asbestos

fibers, the inhalation route is responsible for most if not all of the serious health effects (Fig. 1.12). Effects of asbestos fibers are:

a. *Asbestosis*: Asbestosis is defined as diffuse interstitial fibrosis of the lung as a consequence of exposure to asbestos fiber. Symptoms of asbestosis include dyspnea and cough. Common findings are inspiratory basilar crackles and less commonly, clubbing of the fingers. Functional disturbances can include gas exchange abnormalities, a restrictive pattern and obstructive features due to small airways disease. Asbestosis is generally associated with relatively high exposure levels with radiological signs of parenchymal fibrosis. Diagnosis of asbestosis is done by sputum examination for asbestos body, X-ray chest, pulmonary function test, HRCT, lung biopsy, etc.

b. *Malignant mesothelioma*: Malignant mesothelioma effecting any serosal membrane (pleura and peritoneum) may be induced by asbestos inhalation. Therefor these can produce pleural or peritoneal malignant mesothelioma. Inhaled asbestos fibers mainly blue asbestos (crocidolite) can penetrate the structure in between lung and abdomen and reach peritoneum to develop peritoneal mesothelioma. Mesothelioma is frequently present with pleural effusion, dyspnea, and chest pain.

c. *Lung cancer*: Clinical signs and symptoms of asbestos-related cancer do not differ from those of lung cancer of other causes. The presence of asbestosis is an indicator of high exposure. Asbestosis may also contribute some additional risk of lung cancer beyond that conferred by asbestos exposure alone. The interaction between smoking, asbestos exposure and lung cancer is the best-studied example of the influence of smoking on occupational disease. Studies of asbestos workers indicate a substantially increased risk of lung cancer, and lung cancers occur at greater than additive rates (usually synergistic or multiplication effect) in person exposed to both asbestos and cigarette smoke.

d. *Skin corn or asbestos wart*: Workers with a great deal of unprotected skin contact with asbestos (from handling this material with their bare hands) would sometimes develop nodular skin lesions termed asbestos corns or warts. When asbestos fibers get into the skin as a result of abrasion, they provoke a low-grade inflammatory reaction with hyperkeratosis which eventually swells out, taking the fibers with it and leaving no scar. These benign lesions are a foreign body reaction from fibers embedded in the skin.

3. *Coal workers' pneumoconiosis (CWP)*: Coal is not a pure mineral. It is formed by the accumulation of vegetable matter covered by sedimentary rock to seal it from air and

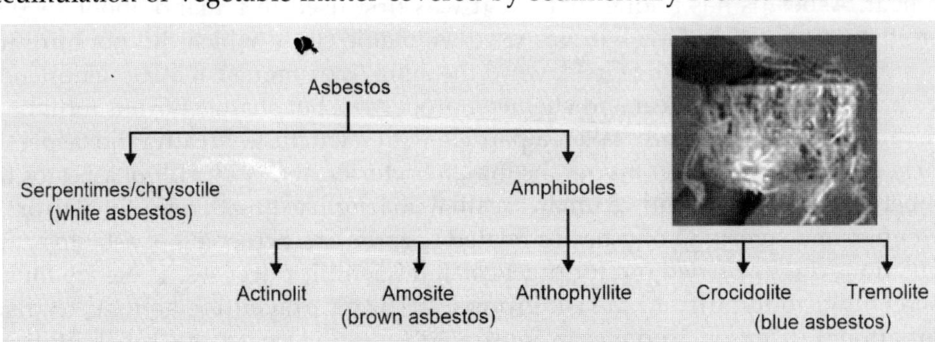

Fig. 1.12: Types of asbestos

subjected to pressure and temperature. It causes the physical and chemical property to change. Coal is comprised of moisture, pure coal (carbon) and mineral matter (mainly sulfur). Coal workers' pneumoconiosis is virtually confined to underground coal-miners, though it may occur in any place where a worker is exposed to high levels of coal dust in poorly ventilated conditions. Thus, it has been described in coal trimmers, loading coal in the holds of ships, and in men and women sorting coal on surface screens. Some other sources of coal/carbon are carbon black and coke.

Effect of Coal Dust Inhalation

a. *Coal-workers' pneumoconiosis (CWP)*: CWP results from the inhalation and deposition of coal mine dust and the lung's reaction to its presence. Typically, CWP is described as simple pneumoconiosis and progressive massive fibrosis (PMF). Simple coal-workers' pneumoconiosis is the early stage of CWP and it is reversible. The miners with simple CWP have no symptoms or sign attributable to the disease. As the disease progresses to PMF, the combination of fibrous masses and associated emphysema leads to increasing breathlessness which is initially on exertion. These lesions may also cavitate and the worker may expectorate an ink-like fluid known as melanoptysis. This stage may progress further till death even though the workers are withdrawn from the exposure. The X-ray findings at the last stage of the disease looks like a typical angel's wings or bat's wings.
b. *Caplan's syndrome*: Caplan's syndrome is a rare condition occurring in dust-exposed workers with rheumatoid diathesis (with or without clinical arthritis).

HEALTH HAZARDS OF METALS AND THEIR COMPOUNDS

'Metal' is a general term referring to elements with a typical lustrous appearance, which the good conductors of heat and electricity and which take part in chemical reactions as positive ions (cations). The 'metal' refers to those elements in the periodic table that have specific characteristics. They are good conductors of heat and electricity; they are bright, shiny and malleable; and they produce a ringing sound when struck. Metals lose electrons to form cations, and the resulting electropositivity gives it an affinity to bind with sulfur, chlorine and other non-metals to form compounds. Alloys are formed from a homogenous mix of metals with other elements. Examples are brass (copper and zinc), bronze (copper and tin), and steel (iron and carbon). These often have physical properties that are different from their components. The term 'superalloys' which has been used for alloys with excellent mechanical strength, and the ability to resist deformation at high temperature. Many superalloys are based on nickel or cobalt. Metaloids are elements, such as antimony, arsenic, polonium and tellurium. They have properties in between those of metals and non-metals.

1. *Lead and its compounds*: Lead is a bluish-grey metal with the symbol Pb, atomic number 82 and atomic weight 207.2. Due to high specific gravity (sg 11.34), ease to casting and fabrication, low melting point (327.4°C), resistance to corrosion and opacity to X-rays, it has had a wide range of uses, such as soldering, printing type, ammunition, brass, piping and shielding against X-rays. Inorganic lead has been used in paint pigments, glass and ceramics. Among organic lead compounds, tetraethyl lead was used extensively as an anti-knocking agent in gasoline. Lead oxide is the most toxic and lead chromate is the least toxic inorganic lead. Tetraethyl lead is the most toxic and tetramethyl lead is the least toxic organic lead. Inhalation is the main route of entry for inorganic lead. Ingestion is often the

principal route of entry, particularly where good standards of personal hygiene are not ingested upon. Lead workers who are allowed to eat or drink in their workplace without first careful washing their hands are unnecessarily increasing the risk they run as are those who smoke at work. Inorganic lead compounds are not significantly absorbed through the skin but organic ones may be. Lead is mainly excreted through the kidneys (75%). Other routes include bile, sweat and the keratinized tissue.

a. *Hazards of inorganic lead*: Classically, the patient with lead poisoning presents with a history of abdominal pain, colic and constipation. Lead is nephrotoxic, cardiotoxic, and central nervous system symptoms including irritability, restlessness, insomnia and other sleep disturbances, fatigue, vertigo, headache, poor memory, tremor, depression, symptoms can progress to drowsiness, stupor, hallucinations, delirium, convulsion and coma. A typical poisoning in adults with lead, the major symptoms and signs are abdominal pain, anemia and muscle weakness (peripheral neuropathy). There may be 'wrist drop' and 'footdrop'. It has reproductive toxicity to both sexes. Another well-known manifestation of lead exposure is a bluish line on the gums. This is so-called Burtonian lead line.

b. *Organic lead*: Mild intoxication is characterized by nervous instability. Common symptoms include insomnia, troubled dreams, emotional instability, and heightened and erratic physical activity. In severe cases, the prodromal stage develops into violent symptoms, sometimes gradually but most often suddenly. These consist of delusions, hallucinations, and hyperactivity, with constant moving, loud shouting, and laughing. The hyperactivity may go on continually for several days before it ends up in coma and death or, alternatively, in recovery. Organic lead can reduce IQ. The biochemical tests include blood lead, urine lead, blood ZPP estimations, etc.

2. *Mercury poisoning*: Mercury (Hg) is a metal that is liquid at room temperature under normal pressure, with a high specific gravity (sg 13.59 at 12°C), high expansion coefficient and large surface tension. Many metals can be mixed with mercury to form amalgams. The various use of mercury includes thermometers, electrical appliances (lamps, switches, and batteries), extracting gold, and the restoration of teeth (dental amalgam). Mercury is present as inorganic and organic compounds. Mercury and its compounds are absorbed in all three routes. Mercury is excreted in the urine and feces and may also be found in sweat, saliva, and breast milk. Acute poisoning usually results from the accidental or deliberate ingestion of mercury compounds and the toxicity include vomiting and abdominal pain may develop and watery diarrhea, hematemesis and then shock cause death. The classic symptoms of chronic mercury poisoning are tremors, gingivitis and erethism (Greek *erethismos* means irritate). The earliest findings are usually gingivitis, hypersalivation (mercurial ptyalism) and an unpleasant, bitter, metallic taste in the mouth. Gingivitis is most marked in those with poor oral hygiene and may be severe enough to cause loosening or loss of teeth. There may be glossitis, pharyngitis and gastritis, tremors and change of handwriting. There may be mercuria lentis and Minamata disease. Minamata disease was first noted at the end of 1953 when an unusual neurological disorder began to affect the villagers living on Minamata Bay on the Southern Coast of the most southernly of the main island of Japan. It was commonly referred to as "kibyo", that is, the mystery illness. It was an outbreak of chronic methyl mercury poisoning due to the ingestion of contaminated fish from the Minamata Bay in Japan.

3. *Arsenic poisoning*: Today, arsenic is employed in metallurgy, agriculture (as a cotton desiccant), animal husbandry (for sheep dip and growth promotion of swine and poultry)

and forestry (as a silvicide). These industrial applications account for the majority of the uses of inorganic and organic arsenic compounds. Arsine (AsH_3) is a colorless gas which is odorless at low concentration but smells of garlic at high concentration. It is formed whenever arsenic comes in contact with nascent pure hydrogen: $As + 3H = AsH_3$. Toxicity may be acute when there is ingestion of inorganic arsenic. It causes acute diarrhea, shock and death. The chronic toxicity usually due to organic arsenic are like hyperpigmentation, eczematous dermatitis, ulceration of skin, skin cancer, loss of vibration sense, difficulty in walking, pain and burning sensation of calf muscles, hepatic cirrhosis, anemia, painless perforation of nasal septa, bronchitis, pneumonitis, broad wide strip type of line under the nailbed called 'mess line'. Arsine gas is the gaseous form of arsenic which is very toxic. It is the commonest cause of occupational jaundice.

4. *Chromium poisoning*: Chromium and its compounds protect against rust, provide color, conserve energy as components of catalysts, prevent decay, resist soiling, and are used in hundreds of other ways, such as in the manufacturing of foam rubber. Chromium is a very complex and versatile metal whose harmful effects are heavily dependent on valence. In addition to metallic chromium (valence 0), other valences found in industry are the +2, +3, +4, +5, and +6 combining states. Trivalent and hexavalent chromium are the only compounds known to be significantly associated with human disease. Hexavalent chromium is most toxic because it can be absorbed through the skin but trivalent cannot. It may cause contact dermatitis, chrome ulcer, perforation of nasal septa, asthma, pneumonitis, conjunctivitis and lungs cancer.
5. *Nickel poisoning*: Nickel is used for the production of stainless steel, nickel alloys, nickel cast iron, alkaline batteries (nickel cadmium batteries), pigments and it is used for electroplating and electroforming. It may cause itching called nickel itch, lungs cancer, cancer of nasal septa, etc. Nickel carbonyl is one of the most toxic within the all toxic metal fumes in industries. It causes lungs alveolar damage and enzyme system damage very quickly.
6. *Cobalt poisoning*: Cobalt (Co) is a silvery-gray, shiny, hard metal. The main route of absorption during occupational exposure is through inhalation. Refined cobalt is available to the industrial market primarily as broken or cut cathodes and to a small extent as electrolytic coarse powder. The toxicities of cobalt are—interstitial fibrosis called hard-metal pneumoconiosis, occupational asthma, cardiomyopathy, allergic dermatitis, affect thyroid gland (increase T4). The international Agency for Research on Cancer (IARC) concluded that cobalt and its compounds are possibly carcinogenic to human.
7. *Aluminum toxicity*: Aluminum is produced from ores (primary production) and scrap (secondary production). Aluminum is a light metal, which is used more widely throughout industry than any other non-ferrous metal. Its major applications are in transportation, building and construction, packaging and electrical equipment. A wide spectrum of respiratory symptoms and diseases, including interstitial fibrosis, pneumoconiosis, occupational asthma, granulomatous disease, chronic obstructive pulmonary disease, emphysema, desquamative interstitial pneumonia, and pulmonary alveolar proteinosis has been described to occupational activities involving exposure to aluminum dust or fumes. In the handling of minerals which contain aluminum (bauxite and corundum), exposure to aluminum accompanied by exposure to silica. This combined exposure may lead to the development of fibrosis of the lung (Shaver's disease). China-clay workers exposing to hydrated aluminum silicate may suffer from the disease known as Kaolinosis. It may cause Alzheimer's disease consists of deterioration of mental function

involving memory, judgement, abstract thinking as well as changes in personality and behavior.

8. *Beryllium poisoning*: Beryllium has chemical and physical properties that make it desirable for high technology applications. The application of beryllium and its alloys are widespread, including use in aerospace, the automotive industries, dental alloys, electronics, computers, nuclear weapons and telecommunications. Exposure to beryllium dust and fumes can cause an immune hypersensitivity reaction, dermatitis and lung diseases, including acute berylliosis, chronic beryllium disease and lung cancer, most hazardous exposures to beryllium come from dust or fume generated by disturbing the surface of a beryllium product through machining and polishing processes.

Occupational Carcinoma

1. *Skin carcinoma*: The causes may be: Coal tars and pitches, X-ray, dyes, certain oils, sunrays, arsenic and arsenic compounds, benzo(a)anthracene, benzo(a)pyrene.
2. *Lungs carcinoma*: The causes may be: Asbestos fiber, free silica dust, nickel, chromium, coal tar, radioactive substances, cigarette smoking, petroleum products, beryllium, cadmium, formaldehyde.
3. *Bladder carcinoma*: The causes may be: Beta-naphthylamine, benzene, para-aminodiphenyl, arsenic.
4. *Blood cancer*: The causes may be: Benzene, ionizing radiation, phenoxy acid herbicides and dioxins, some chlorinated organic compounds.

Occupational Dermatitis

- *Physical agents*, e.g.
  - a. Heat
  - b. Cold
  - c. Moisture
  - d. Friction
  - e. Pressure
  - f. X-ray.
- *Chemical agents*, e.g.
  - a. Acid
  - b. Alkali
  - c. Dyes
  - d. Solvent
  - e. Grease, tar and pitch
  - f. Chlorinated phenols.
- *Biological agents*, e.g.
  - a. Living agents:
    - i. Viruses
    - ii. Bacteria
    - iii. Fungi
    - iv. Parasites.
  - b. Plant products
    - i. Leaves
    - ii. Vegetables

iii. Fruits
iv. Flowers
v. Vegetable dust.

EXPOSURE OF TOXIC AGENTS IN FIRE HAZARD

The main threats to life in fires are toxic gases, heat and oxygen deficiency. The temperature in a room in a house fire can easily reach 500–1000°C, and as many as 400 toxic compounds can be demonstrated in the smoke. The principal toxic constituents of smoke are soot, carbon monoxide, carbon dioxide, nitrogen oxides, hydrogen cyanide, hydrogen chloride, sulfur dioxide, hydrogen fluoride, hydrogen sulfide, isocyanates, acrolein, benzene, phenol, formaldehyde and a range of chlorinated hydrocarbons. Carbon monoxide is an important factor in 50–80% of all fire fatalities. The role of hydrogen cyanide is less clear, although it is formed in many fires especially those involving wool, silk, nylon and polyurethane products. The chemistry involved in combustion reactions is extremely complex, even in the simplest example, such as the burning of jet of natural gas or methane in oxygen or air, when numerous reactive species, including free radicals (such as OH, O and CH_3) are produced which eventually form mainly carbon dioxide, water and large particles of carbon (soot).

$$CH_4 + 2O_2 = CO_2 + 2H_2O$$

Smoke comprises a mixture of gases, liquid and solid particles which arises as combustion and pyrolysis products. Predicting the products of combustion (oxidative degeneration) and pyrolysis (thermal decomposition) of burning materials and hence determining in retrospect the effects of exposure of fireman or other victims to the constituents of a smoke plume is not straightforward. Some general principles can be considered. Materials consumed by fires contain carbon, hydrogen and oxygen as their main elements, and hence the bulk of all combustion products will consist of compounds formed from these, e.g. carbon monoxide and carbon dioxide. The next important elements are halogens (mostly chlorine) and nitrogen, with smaller amounts of elements such as sulfur and phosphorus. Almost all the inorganic anions are released as the irritant acid gases, hydrogen chloride and hydrogen fluoride, if fluorine is present. For the nitrogen present in well-ventilated fires oxides of nitrogen are released, but in large fires in buildings, where the ventilation is poorer, a larger proportion of the nitrogen is released as hydrogen cyanide. Organic compounds may form a number of partially decomposed products, e.g. formaldehyde, acrolein, and crotonaldehyde and possibly free radicals that add to the irritancy of the smoke. Other compounds, such as decomposition products from isocyanates, styrene and phenol, may also be important. Fires in warehouses storing chemicals will potentially release a cocktail of irritants and toxic substances which may greatly add to the hazard of the fire plume.

Polyvinyl chloride (PVC) is the most widely used plastic and fires involving large amounts of this material at storage sites and recycling installations are not uncommon and attract notoriety because they are difficult for the fire services to put out while they generate toxic plumes. At over 300°C, PVC decomposes to form hydrogen chloride and carbon monoxide together with small amounts of about 50 various hydrocarbons. About 50% of the polymer's weight comes off as hydrogen chloride, and the irritancy of the plume is added to by the presence of acrolein, ammonia, sulfur dioxide, nitrogen dioxide, aldehydes and particles. Phosgene is produced only in rare circumstances. There is no doubt that dioxins are formed whenever chlorinated plastics are burned: in a large-scale plastics fire typically involving 500–1000 tons of PVC as much as 1–2 kg of dioxins could be produced.

When there is fire in a naturally pressurized oil well, the plume contained carbon dioxide, carbon monoxide, sulfur dioxide and particles, including soot. The major health concern revolved around the particle fallout that contained elemental carbon, rock/soil particles, metal oxides, silicates, vanadium, nickel and polycyclic aromatic hydrocarbons besides smoke rained oil drops.

The products released the combustion of wood are more difficult to measure mainly because the tendency for some to incinerate more rapidly at high temperature. The occupational health of forest firefighters and the workers who manage fire are at great risks. The number of possible products of vegetation combustion is almost limitless and every fuel and condition of vegetation burning products a unique pattern. It is possible and practical to select a limit number of by-products that are most likely to be involved in the acute toxicity of smoke. Two of the most important are formaldehyde and acrolein. Both appear to occur in all smoke. The toxicology of both is well studied, they are powerful respiratory irritants. There seems to be a reasonable prospect that free radical precursors with half-lives in the tens of the minutes are produced when cellulosic materials burn. If so, they will reach the respiratory pulmonary cells. Ozone is not produced in the fire, but the various hydrocarbons of smoke are substrates for reactions that eventually produce ozone, and that production may continue for miles down-plume. The effects of best-known component are particulate matters.

Air emissions from open tyre fires have been shown to be more toxic (e.g. mutagenic) than those of a combustor, regardless of the fuel. Open tire fire emissions include 'criteria' pollutants, such as particulates, carbon monoxide (CO), sulfur dioxides (SO_2), oxides of nitrogen (NOx), and volatile organic compounds (VOCs). They also include "non-criteria" hazardous air pollutants (HAPs), such as polynuclear aromatic hydrocarbons (PAHs), dioxins, furans, hydrogen chloride, benzene, polychlorinated biphenyls (PCBs); and metals such as arsenic, cadmium, nickel, zinc, mercury, chromium, and vanadium. Both criteria and HAP emissions from an open tyre fire can represent significant acute (short-term) and chronic (long-term) health hazards to firefighters and nearby residents. Depending on the length and degree of exposure, these health effects could include irritation of the skin, eyes, and mucous membranes, respiratory effects, central nervous system depression, and cancer. Firefighters and others working near a large tyre fire should be equipped with respirators and dermal protection. Unprotected exposure to the visible smoke plume should be avoided.

Toxicity resulting from the massive use of plastics in our modern society is not restricted to exposures sustained by workers during synthesis, formulation, or manufacture. Rapid and nearly complete oxidation of plastic products occurs with the application of extreme heat during a conflagration, resulting in carbon dioxide, water and oxide of nitrogen. Even so, partially degraded molecules result, and these may recombine to form new molecular species. Thermal degradation often begins at relatively low temperature (200–400°C), producing hydrogen chloride, carbon dioxide, carbon monoxide, and some hydrocarbons. Neoprenes release sulfur dioxide and hydrogen sulfide. Rigid urathanes and isocyanates also produce CO_2, CO and small amount of $CFCl_3$, HCN, HCl and hydrocarbons. Although the expected toxicity results from those compounds released in greater amounts, those emitted in smaller amounts cannot be disregarded for two major reasons:

a. They are very toxic (e.g. benzene and hydrogen cyanide)
b. Certain workers are hypersusceptible for some reasons, e.g. allergy to isocyanates and pharmacobiochemical sensitivity as encountered occasionally with amines and certain halogenated hydrocarbons.

Not only should the major parent compounds be considered but also additives, such as accelerators, catalysts, copolymers, dyes, fillers, mold lubricants, pigments, plasticizers, solvents, stabilizers, and ultraviolet absorbers. There are a number of syndromes being reported that appear to result from thermal degradation products of plastics.

Teflon fume fever has been reported, especially in smokers exposed to teflon fume generated by temperatures far in excess of those achieved during the cooking with teflon coated utensils.

Meat wrapper's asthma is another alleged syndrome that appears to be associated with exposure to heated plastics, in this instance, hot wire cutting of polyvinyl chloride film. There are instances of adverse reactions when urethane foams, polystyrene, and other plastics are thermally degraded.

Fire in a pressurized tunnel burns more intensely for a given flame size, spreads more vigorously and is harder to extinguish than atmospheric pressure and all of these effects are magnified by oxygen enrichment. So, the fire risk depends on both pressure and percentage of oxygen in the environment and remains a major safety consideration in compressed air work.

Classification of Fire

1. Class 'A' fire (ordinary fire): Fire in ordinary combustible materials such as wood, paper, etc.
2. Class 'B' fire (oil substances fire): Fire in flammable liquid like petrol, diesel, etc.
3. Class 'C' fire (gas fire): Fire involving gaseous substances under pressure like liquid petroleum gas, etc.
4. Class 'D' fire (metal fire): Fire involving metals.
5. Class 'E' fire: Fire involving electrical equipment.

EFFECTS OF OXYGEN DEFICIENCY

Oxygen-deficient atmosphere can be encountered in mines, and other underground or confined spaces. The main danger of suddenly entering an atmosphere devoid of oxygen is that it will lead to an almost immediate loss of consciousness without warning; even very quiet breathing will produce sudden loss of consciousness within 50 seconds when all the remaining oxygen in the lungs has gone.

It is the partial pressure of oxygen, not its percentage, which is of physiological importance, but gas measuring instruments and alarms record volume concentrations. A drop of 3–4% of oxygen by volume is a little physiological significance in humans, but it will extinguish a candle flame. The level of oxygen has to fall to 13% volume before symptoms become very noticeable.

The effects of low oxygen concentration are as follows:

1. 16–13%: Dizziness and shortness of breath on exertion; pulse rate accelerated and volume of breathing increased. Ability to maintain attention is diminished but it can be restored with conscious mental effort.
2. 13–10%: Judgment faulty. Rapid fatigue and fainting on exertion. Severe injuries cause no pain. Emotional lability.
3. 10–6%: Nausea and vomiting. Loss of ability to perform any vigorous muscular movements or even to move at all.
4. < 6%: Loss of consciousness with fainting or coma. Rapidly fatal.

Confined Spaces

Working in enclosed spaces with inadequate natural ventilation is a well-known cause of death from asphyxia due to oxygen deficiency or from a build-up of toxic gases and vapors, such as carbon monoxide, carbon dioxide, methane, ammonia, hydrogen sulfide, petroleum vapor and liquid petroleum gas. The examples of confined spaces are: trenches, pits, sewers, tunnels, submarines and spacecraft. Toxic substances are accumulated where workers are welding or flame-cutting. In addition, the presence of flammable gases such as butane, propane and petrol, all of which are normally heavier than air, can be responsible for explosions in tanks. The risk of fire and explosion may be increased by enrichment of the air by oxygen in the event of a leak from an oxygen cylinder forming part of welding equipment. Oxygen deficiency in pits can arise from an ingress of methane or absorption of oxygen by certain constituents of soil. The rotting of vegetation and the rusting of metalwork inside tanks also consume oxygen. Manholes, tunnels and trenches in limestone soil can partly fill with carbon dioxide formed by the action of acid groundwater. Apparently safe atmospheres can become suddenly dangerous if the residues and sludges in tanks or in sewers are disturbed by the worker walking in them, or by water surges following sudden heavy rainfall. In construction industry, pipe-freezing work is carried out using liquid nitrogen to solidify soil to enable drilling to be performed in wet conditions and fatalities have occurred from the cold gas pushing out the available air.

In order to avoid gassing accidents, safe systems of work must be adhered to and these often require the use of electronic monitors or detector tubes to test for toxic, flammable and asphyxiating gases before initial entry to a confined space and while the work continues. The space should be well ventilated before entry; otherwise, appropriate breathing apparatus has to be worn.

HEALTH HAZARDS OF METAL ARC WELDING IN INDUSTRY

Metal welding is a genetic term for any of the processes, ubiquitous in industry, of joining metals at areas or point softened or liquefied by the application of heat, sometime with associated local pressure.

The toxic agents responsible for health hazards:

A. *Particulate emission*: Two main groups of particulates may be emitted from electric arc welding process:
   1. Fractioned mixed metal oxide particles are formed from metal which is vaporized in the high temperature of the arc and then condensed, often reacting with oxygen in the air, to form chain and aggregates reflecting the composition of the electrode but with the more volatile constituents predominately. The most of these particles are in the respirable range, e.g. iron, zinc, aluminum, cadmium, and chromium.
   2. The second group of particles is term 'spatter'. These are coarser, discreet, unfractionated particles of electrode, usually larger than the respirable range.

B. *Gaseous emission*: The principal gases are:
   1. Ozone
   2. Oxide of nitrogen
   3. CO

C. Heat

D. Noise.

Health Effects

Respiratory System

1. *Acute effect*:
   a. *Asphyxia*: When working in an inadequately ventilated confined space where oxygen has been displaced by inert shielding gases or depleted by combustion or rusting of ferrous structures.
   b. *Inhalation fever*: The term inhalation fever collectively describes as a group of acute, non-allergic, usually benign and self-limiting flue-like illness caused by heavy exposure to certain inhalable environmental pollutant. The most common of these is metal fumes fever, with polymer fumes fever.

   Metal fumes fever: It is one of the few ancient occupational diseases still encountered in modern industrial practice, is quite common among welders, the percentage reporting an attack when asked specifically has been variously reported as 10% and 30%. It is an unpleasant but uncomplicated, self-limiting, non-allergic, influenza-like reaction following a single exposure to high concentration of metal fumes. The syndrome consisting of fever, chills, muscle pains and malaise, generally with relatively mild respiratory symptoms, and classically little or no radiographic or functional abnormalities, although this is not always the case. The symptoms usually begin a few hours after a heavy exposure to metal oxides and they subside spontaneously after 24 hours or night's sleep. Zinc fume fever commonly occurs, e.g. after the smelting or thermal spraying of zinc without adequate exhaust, or after welding or flame cutting galvanized steel in a confined space. No specific treatment is required, except preventive hygiene measures.
2. *Chronic health effect*:
   a. Chronic bronchitis:
      - More in smokers
      - There is dose-response relationship.
   b. Occupational asthma

   It may be caused by inhalation of irritants or sensitizing agents, e.g. nickel, chromium, iron, and zinc.

Central and Peripheral Nervous System

1. Neuropsychiatric symptoms in aluminum toxicity
2. Manganese toxicity.

Reproductive System

Welding may cause reduction of fertility due to:

1. Exposure to radiant heat
2. Exposure to metal like chromium, nickel, manganese, and cadmium.

Physical Injury

Musculoskeletal system injury like accident, injury, shoulder pain, and low back pain.

Skin

1. Ray burn
2. Permanent pigmentation in the unprotected areas of skin

3. Welding may affect the exposed skin in other ways like siderosis
4. Contact dermatitis
5. Photodermatitis.

Ear and Hearing

1. Burn inside the ear is uncommon but very painful
2. Perforation of tympanic membrane with deafness
3. Facial paralysis
4. High rate of residual and recurrent perforation
5. NIHL.

Eyes

1. Eye injury from foreign body.
2. Arc-eye due to exposure of arc's ultraviolet radiation. Arc eye is an acute high flux ultraviolet injury to the corneal epithelium causing a punctuate superficial keratitis in the welder whose eyes have not been adequately protected when he has struck the electric arc to begin welding. Some injuries are caused by reflected radiation. It is also known as flash eye. Typical presentation after 4–5 hours like:
   a. Pain due to spasm of iris and ciliary muscles
   b. Photophobia
   c. Excess lacrimation
   d. Feeling of grittiness or foreign body sensation.

   The eyes will be normal if take rest for 48 hours.

Cardiovascular System

1. The toxic effect of soluble barium in fumes from certain filler wires and consumable electrodes shown to be cardiotoxic.
2. Electromagnetic field can develop disturbances to the pacemaker.

Welding fumes cannot be classified simply. The composition and quantity of both are dependent on the alloy being welded and the process and electrodes used. Reliable analysis of fumes cannot be made without considering the nature of the welding process and system being examined; reactive metals and alloys such as aluminum and titanium are arc-welded in a protective, inert atmosphere such as argon. These arcs create relatively little fume, but an intense radiation which can produce ozone. Similar processes are used to arc-weld steels, also creating a relatively low level of fumes. Ferrous alloys also are arc-welded in oxidizing environments which generate considerable fume, and can produce carbon monoxide instead of ozone. Such fumes generally are composed of discrete particles of amorphous slags containing iron, manganese, silicon and other metallic constituents depending on the alloy system involved. Chromium and nickel compounds are found in fumes when stainless steels are arc-welded. Some coated and flux-cored electrodes are formulated with fluorides and the fumes associated with them can contain significantly more fluorides than oxides. Because of the above factors, arc-welding fumes frequently must be tested for individual constituents which are likely to be present to determine whether specific TLVs are exceeded. Conclusions based on total fume concentration are generally adequate if no toxic elements are present in welding rod, metal coating and conditions are not conducive to the formation of toxic gases.

The following preventive measures must be taken to achieve adequate control of the welding hazards:

1. Prevent emission by selection/substitution of process; improve working practices by modification of process, process parameters or consumables to lower fume and gas emission rates or toxicity of the constituents.
2. Prevent exposure by natural ventilation and/or engineering controls, including isolation or segregation, control of pollutants at the source by the local exhaust ventilation.
3. Prevent exposure by wearing personal protective equipment.

OCCUPATIONS INVOLVING RISK OF CONTAINING THESE OCCUPATIONAL DISEASES

A. *Effects of work on health*: Work can affect health in several ways, like:

1. Occupational exposure may be a direct cause of ill health, e.g. exposure to hydrogen cyanide gas encountered by firefighters during their work can cause cyanide poisoning.
2. Occupational exposure, while not necessarily being the sole factor causing disease and be one of a number of contributory causes. Cigarette smoking multiplies the risk for lung cancer if there is exposure to asbestos fibers or radon gas. Each of these can cause lung cancer independently, but a worker who smokes, lives in a high environment radon area or is exposed to asbestos from work activities has a much-increased risk of lung cancer. Another example is that of exposure to carbon monoxide which can result from smoking, following exposure to methylene chloride (used as a paint stripper), and working in an enclosed space like garage which is heated by a gas-fire heater, and has a car engine running. All these factors act independently to increase blood carboxyhemoglobin, but when several of these sources of carbon monoxide are present there, there is an elevated risk of carbon monoxide poisoning.
3. The nature of job may worsen pre-existing non-occupational disease. Hairdressing producer or working in kitchen can result in a worsening of endogenous eczema.
4. The occupational environment may give easy access to potentially harmful materials, increasing the risk of their abuse. Adverse health effects resulting from availability to toxic agents are effects of anesthetic gases in anesthetists or other health care staffs or suicide in farm workers using pesticides.

B. *Effects of health on work*: Following a period of sickness absence, it is in a patient's and society's interest to encourage a return to work. Many people with some impairment of function either seek work or seek to remain at work. This may affect his work by the following ways:

1. The patient's condition may limit, reduce or prevent him performing the job effectively, e.g. the musculoskeletal conditions that reduce mobility or diminish manipulative ability.
2. The patient's condition might be made worse by the job (excessive physical exertion in some cardiorespiratory condition).
3. The patient's condition is likely to make it unsafe to do the job (liability to sudden loss of consciousness while working alone and at height).
4. The patient's condition is obviously/likely to make it unsafe for third parties, such as coworkers, visitors or members of the public, e.g. a bus or train driver who is prone to

episode of unconsciousness with no warning symptoms may cause an accident affecting other crew members, passengers and public.

5. The patient's condition might make it unsafe for the community (for consumer of a product, if a food-handler transmits infection).

Correlation Between Environmental Exposure and Health Status

The main factors which regulate the occupational health status are:

1. Nature of substance of exposure.
2. Intensity or severity of exposure.
3. Length of exposure.
4. Personal susceptibility.
5. Quantum of exposure.
6. *Bioavailability*: The bioavailability of a toxic substance indicates the extent of which the agent reaches the site of action. If it is not in bioavailable form, as in the case with many orally ingested toxic substances that cause vomiting or diarrhea, it will be removed promptly. In other cases, some of the agents will be inactivated before it reaches the site of action, e.g. when cyanide is taken orally, it is absorbed and passes to the liver, where the enzyme rhodanese may metabolize a portion of the ingested cyanide. On the other hand, if the cyanide in the form of gaseous hydrocyanic acid (HCN) is absorbed through the pulmonary circulation, it goes directly to the brain, where it may cause damage from hypoxia.

MODE OF CAUSATION OF OCCUPATIONAL DISEASES AND ITS EFFECTS

The main routes of entry of toxic materials are:

1. *Inhalation*: Inhalation by far the most important route of intake of airborne contaminants. In an industrial environment various substance, solid, liquid or gases are therein the air. In the process of breathing, these airborne contaminants come in the contact with the respiratory system. The respiratory system serves as the portal of entry into the body for a great variety of airborne substances, both gaseous and particulate matters. Many of these contaminants are capable of producing injury and diseases when they are deposited and accumulated in sufficient amount in the lungs or after transfer from the lung in sensitive sites deeper within the body.

   For all particles, a major determining characteristic of the behavior of the particle in the respiratory tract is the size. Size is measured not by geometric dimensions but by sedimentation. The 'aerodynamic diameter' of a particle is what the diameter would be of a perfect sphere sedimenting at the same velocity, correcting for density. Particles above 10 μm aerodynamic diameter tend to be deposited in the nose and larger airways due to inertial impaction. Particles with an aerodynamic diameter <10 μm but >5 μm attain sufficient inertia to become trapped in the smaller airways and at bronchial bifurcation. Particles (little particles) of <0.5 μm in diameter may either remain airborne and be exhaled or be pushed into the mucosa because of the phenomenon of brownian movement. They are kept aloft by molecular motion (heat) 'nudging' them from all sides. They also may be cleared by the process of phagocytosis. Thus, the particles in the midrange are most likely to penetrate to the alveoli and, once there, to sediment and to deposit on the airspace wall. This so-called 'respiratory range' between about 0.5 μm and 5 μm is a primary concern in the inhalation of particulates. They are known as respirable dust.

2. *Through skin*: Many gaseous and liquid materials are absorbed to a limited extent through the intact skin. When this occurs, the predominant action may be local, at the point of contact, or systemic. The amount of skin absorption generally is proportionate to the surface area of contact and to the lipid solubility of the toxic agents. Phenol, cresol, nitrobenzene, aniline, TEL, parathion, etc. may pose a great hazard through skin absorption than through inhalation. Absorption of solid materials through skin is not common. Absorption of toxic chemicals through skin is more through abraded than intact skin.
3. *Ingestion*: It may result from many sources like contaminated food and smoking. It is the least important rout of absorption in occupational scenario. The amount of absorption through GI tract is usually proportionate to the gastrointestinal surface area and its blood flow and depends on the physical state of the agent. Most toxic agents are absorbed in the small intestine.
4. *Ocular absorption*: Toxic chemical can also be absorbed through eyes. Eyes are also the site of absorption. When the chemicals enter the body through the conjunctiva, they bypass the hepatic circulation and are responsible for severe systemic toxicity. This may occur when the organophosphate pesticides are splashed into the eyes.

Metabolism of Toxic Chemicals

Absorption and Distribution of Chemicals

Foreign or exogenous chemical (xenobiotics) must be absorbed from the surrounding environment and transported to their target site in the body for a toxic effect to occur. The chemical has to cross the many cell membranes which form a lipoprotein barrier to the outside as well as maintain the integrity of the cell. The specific transport mechanisms that have evolved are to facilitate the absorption and distribution of nutrients rather than toxic chemicals. Consequently, most xenobiotics are transported by simple methods and not complex carrier-associated processes. A carrier for an endogenous substance unless the xenobiotic compounds have a very similar structure it will not usually be able to bind to the carrier. Lipid solubility is one of the major factors determining the extent and rate of simple diffusion through a lipoprotein membrane. Lipophilic molecules diffuse more readily than those that are hydrophilic, the rate of transport being dependent on the partition coefficient (the ratio of solubility in octane/water).

Toxicokinetic

The investigation and management of a patient exposed to toxic chemicals requires at least a basic knowledge of the concept of toxicokinetic alongside an understanding of the mechanism by which chemicals gain entry to the body and are biotransformed into nontoxic or occasionally, toxic metabolites. Toxicokinetic is the study of dynamic (kinetic) relationships between the concentration of a chemical (toxicon) in body fluids and tissues and its biological effects. Toxicokinetic analysis produces a mathematical description of the dynamics of absorption, distribution and elimination of chemical. Although involving the descriptive use of mathematical value in that the understanding can be uses to evaluate the significance of blood concentrations in biological monitoring and to determine the nature of exposure control (risk management).

Most toxic xenobiotics have no nutritional value and are metabolized primarily to reduce potential toxicity and facilitate their elimination from the body. The majority of compounds that gain entry most easily to the body are lipophilic and likely, therefore, to be retained and before they can be excreted must be converted into a form that is more easily eliminated. The liver is the major organ for the metabolism (biotransformation) of such compound. The principal function of biotransformation is to facilitate the elimination of a foreign agent by its conversion to a more polar (water soluble) metabolite and is therefore, a detoxification mechanism and then it is more readily excreted in the urine.

Toxic substances are excreted either unchanged or as metabolites. Excretory organs other than lungs eliminate polar (water-soluble) compounds more efficiently than no-polar (lipid-soluble) compounds. The kidney is the primary organ of elimination for most polar compounds and their metabolites. Many toxic substances metabolized by the liver are excreted first in the bile and later eliminated in the stool and reabsorbed into the blood. Some toxic substances may be excreted through saliva, breast milk, and there may be some minor removal in hair or skin. The volatile gases are readily excreted by the lung through passive diffusion from the blood, crossing the alveolar-capillary barrier in 'reverse' direction.

DIAGNOSTIC METHODS OF OCCUPATIONAL DISEASES

Occupational diseases are caused by a pathological adaptation of the patient to his working environment; therefore, in order to properly diagnose occupational diseases, one must evaluate both patient and environmental exposure. Very few occupational diseases present with specific pathognomic, clinical, or laboratory findings. Thus, the anemia of benzene intoxication, the peripheral neuritis of acrylamide poisoning, asthma of byssinosis, the fibrosis of asbestosis, the granuloma of berylliosis, the nodulation of silicosis cannot be adequately diagnosed as to etiological agent from clinical and laboratory findings alone. Only with knowledge of exposure, in addition to clinical factors, can an accurate diagnosis be made. Obtaining adequate environmental data and weighing their importance as causative factors can be an extremely difficult problem, especially for one not experience in this.

One should utilize the same process use in the diagnosis of condition, namely, history of symptomatology, past history, family history, and review of the symptoms.

The physical examination should include a general examination, with special emphasis on the organ system likely to be seen in the disease under investigation, e.g. the lead line (blue line) of gum in inorganic lead intoxication, the enlarged liver seen with overexposure to toluene, or the enlarge spleen in overexposure to benzene. Evaluation of exposure, which is necessary in diagnosing work-related conditions, adds a dimension to occupational medicine usually not found in other clinical practice.

Components of a Thorough Occupational History

1. Present job description and nature of work.
2. Hours of work and description of shifts system.
3. Types of workplace hazards:
    a. Physical
    b. Chemical
    c. Biological
    d. Mechanical
    e. Psychosocial.

4. Degree of exposure:
    a. Duration of exposure
    b. Exposure concentration
    c. Route of exposure
    d. Presence and efficacy of exposure controls
    e. Qualitative exposure data from inspections and monitoring.
5. Previous occupations:
    a. Lifetime history, with date of employment and job duties
    b. Hobbies and avocational exposures
    c. Sports.
6. Other jobs or 'Moonlighting'.
7. Time relation between job and symptoms:
    a. Symptoms occur or are exacerbated at work and improve away from work.
    b. Symptoms coincide with the introduction of new exposure at work.
    c. Symptoms coincide with other change in working conditions.
8. Previous significant medical history:
    a. Past illness
    b. Past injury
    c. Past surgery.
9. Presence of an occupational health program at work:
    a. Periodical health surveillance
    b. Workplace environmental assessment
    c. Regulation of workplace exposure
    d. Availability of trained medical and nursing care.
10. Workplace protection:
    a. Use of personal protective equipment on the job.
    b. Methods of material handling.
    c. Engineering protective measures.
11. First aid or acute care provided at the time of injury or illness.
12. Similar complaints among other workers.
13. Presence of any abnormal circumstances at work:
    a. Breakdown or shutdown machines or processes.
    b. Increase demand for production.
    c. Change in personnel, materials or processes.
14. Other environmental exposure:
    a. Home environment
    b. Indoor air quality
    c. Social lifestyle
    d. Smoking habits
    e. Alcohol use
    f. Drug use
    g. Addictive behaviors.

Need of Occupational History

The two main reasons why an occupational history is important:

1. Because of the effects of work on health: Occupational exposures may be a direct cause of ill health, e.g. exposure to hydrogen cyanide gas encountered by firefighters during their work can cause cyanide poisoning, or exposure to metallic mercury in gold miners, or in dentists causes mercury poisoning.
2. Because of the effects of health on the safe and efficient performance of work: The patient's condition may limit, reduce or prevent him performing the job effectively like musculo-skeletal conditions that reduce mobility or diminish manipulative ability or patient's condition is likely to make it unsafe to do the job like liability to sudden loss of consciousness while working alone and at heights.

Laboratory tests done in connection with the occupational disease workup are in five categories:

1. *Tests for general assessment of health and to rule out other conditions*: Evaluation in cases of suspected intoxication should routinely include complete blood count, chest X-ray, electrocardiogram, urine analysis.
2. *Nonspecific tests of exposure*: These nonspecific tests of exposure include mean corpuscular volume, mean corpuscular hemoglobin concentration in case of exposure to hemotoxic agents, aspartate amino transferase (AST-SGOT), alanine amino transferase (ALT-SGPT) in exposure to liver toxins, a reduction in force expiratory volume in 1 second (FEV_1) of pulmonary function test (PFT) during the course of the working day when the patient is exposed to pulmonary irritants, delta aminolevulinic acid in red cells in inorganic lead intoxication.
3. *Tests for the agent or its metabolite that indicate exposure*: There are a number of these tests based on a knowledge of metabolism of the substance involved, e.g. it is known that gradual absorption of inorganic lead is characterized by increased lead in the blood. Exposure to toluene may be detected by analysis of hippuric acid in the urine and exposure to trichloroethylene by trichloroacetic acid in the urine and by breath analysis for the substance itself.
4. *Tests of genetic or acquired susceptibility*: There are an increasing number of tests that establish a susceptibility to a disease condition that may be stimulated, precipitated, or aggravated by occupational exposure. Some of these are as follows:
   a. Hereditary serum α_1 antitrypsin deficiency and chronic obstructive pulmonary diseases.
   b. Glucose-6-phosphate dehydrogenase deficiency and hypersusceptibility to hemolytic chemicals.
   c. Diaphorase deficiency and susceptibility to nitrite exposure.
   d. Immunologic screening tests (IgE, IgG) for hypersensitivity to organic compounds.
5. *Chromosomal alteration*: The rapidly expanding science identifies genetic injury from exposure to physical and chemical agents.

METHODS OF PREVENTION

The various measures for the prevention of occupational diseases may be grouped under four heads: Medical measures, engineering measures, statutory or legislation measures and administrative measures.

Medical Measures

1. *Pre-employment medical examination*: Pre-employment medical examination is done at the time of employment and includes the worker's family, occupational and social history, a thorough physical examination, biological and radiological examinations. The purpose of pre-employment medical examination is to place the right person in the right job and to preserve the data for further comparison.

Hazards	*Undesirable condition*
a. Lead	Anemia, hypertension, nephritis, peptic ulcer
b. Dyes	Skin, bladder and kidney diseases, asthma, precancerous lesion

2. *Periodic medical examination*: The slow development of some occupational diseases is very often, leads to their non-recognition in the early stages and this is harmful to the worker. Therefore, for early diagnosis of occupational diseases periodic medical examination is essential.
   The frequency and content of periodic medical examination will depend upon the type of occupational exposure. Ordinarily workers are examined once in a year. But in certain occupational exposure like lead, toxic dyes, and radium exposures monthly or 6-monthly examinations are indicated. Sometimes, even daily examination may be needed when irritant chemical like dichromate is handled.
3. *Pre-placement medical examination*: This medical examination is done when the worker is shifted from one hazardous area to another hazardous area within the same factory.
4. *Fitness-for-duty examination*: A fitness-for-duty examination is essentially the same evaluation and follows the same rules as a pre-placement examination. The only difference is that a fitness-for-duty examination determines whether a previously hired employee who was able to perform the essential functions of the job is still able to perform these essential functions safely. Ideally, a fitness-for-duty evaluation will determine whether an employee is able to perform his or her duties in a safe and effective manner.
5. *Pre-retirement medical examination*: Pre-retirement medical examination is done to the workers before the retirement to see the health condition at the time of retirement and these records are to be preserved in some occupations, like asbestos and silica prone industries.
6. *Special medical examination*: This medical examination is done in case of long-standing absent.
7. *Medical and health care services*: Occupational health service (OHS).
8. *First-aid center or ambulance room*: The ambulance room shall be separate from the rest of the factory and shall be used only for the purpose of first-aid treatment and rest. According to the Occupational Safety, Health and Working Condition Code, 2020 (Chapter VI), ambulance room in every factory, mine, building or other construction work wherein >500 workers are ordinarily employed.
9. *First-aid box*: There shall in every factory be provided and maintained so as to be readily accessible during all working hours first-aid boxes or cupboard equipped with the prescribed contents, and the number of such boxes or cupboards to be provided and maintained shall not be <1 for every 150 workers ordinarily employed at anyone time in the factory (Section 45 of Factories Act, 1948: First-aid appliances). According to the Occupational Safety, Health and Working Condition Code, 2020 (Chapter VI), adequate first-aid boxes or cupboards with contents readily accessible during all working hours.

10. *Industrial hospital*: As referral center.
11. *ESI scheme*: Employees' State Insurance (ESI) is a self-financing social security and health insurance scheme for Indian workers.
12. *Notification of notifiable occupational diseases*: National Laws and Regulations (According to the Occupational Safety, Health and Working Condition Code, 2020) require the notification of some cases and suspected cases of occupational diseases and these occupational diseases are called 'notifiable occupational diseases'. These diseases are recognized internationally for the purpose of workmen's compensation. The main purpose of notification in industry is to initiate measure for prevention and protection and ensuring their effective application and to investigate the working condition and other circumstances which have caused or suspected to have cause occupational diseases. There is a list of 29 diseases is included as notifiable occupational diseases as per Schedule III and Section 12 of this Code and recognized for the purpose of workmen's compensation as per the Workmen's Compensation Act, 1923. According to this OSH&WC, 2020, Section 12(1), where any worker in an establishment contracts any disease specified in the Third Schedule, the employer of the establishment shall send notice thereof to such authorities, and in such forms and within such time, as may be prescribe by the appropriate government.
13. *Supervision of work environment*: The information that may be obtained during a site visit includes a detailed description of the work process, prior results of industrial hygiene sampling and medical surveillance, list of toxic or hazardous materials used and, most important, a guided tour of the work site with a focus on the specific work areas where the patient has been working.
14. To supervise/acquainted with physical, chemical, biological, mechanical and psychosocial hazards.
15. *To study occupational physiology*: Fatigue and weight carried.
16. *To supervised night-work and shift work.*
17. *To advise on matter connected with health and welfare.*
18. *Maintenance and analysis of records.*
19. *Health education and counseling.*

Engineering Measures

1. *Design of building*: Measures for the prevention of occupational disease should commence in the blueprint stage. The type of floor, wall, height, ceiling, roof, doors, windows, cubic space, and color should receive attention.
2. *Good housekeeping*: It covers general cleanliness, ventilation, lighting, washing, food arrangements and general maintenance. It is a fundamental requirement for the control of occupational diseases.
3. *General ventilation*: There should be efficient exhaust ventilation in the room where dust, gas, and fumes are generated to decrease the airborne contaminants.
4. *Mechanization*: The plant should be mechanized to the fullest possible extent to reduce the hazard of contact with harmful substances.
5. *Substitution*: By substitution is meant the replacement of a harmful material by a harmless one or one of lesser toxicity, e.g. zinc or iron-based paints in place of lead-based paints and acetone or toluene can be used in place of benzene.

6. *Dust control*: Dust can be controlled at the point of origin by water spray (wet method or hydroblasting).
7. *Enclosure*: Enclosure the harmful materials and processes will prevent the escape of dust and fumes into the factory atmosphere.
8. *Isolation*: Sometime it may be necessary to isolate the offensive process in a separate building so that workers not directly connected with the operation are not exposed to the hazards.
9. *Local exhaust ventilation*: By providing local exhaust ventilation, dusts, fumes and other injurious substances can be trapped and extracted 'at source' before they escape into the factory atmosphere. The heart of local exhaust ventilation is the hood which is place as near as possible to the point of origin of the dust or fumes. In this way, the breathing zone of workers may be kept free of dangerous dust and poisonous fumes.
10. *Protection devices*: To provide respiratory and non-respiratory personal protective equipment (PPE).
11. *Environmental monitoring*: To maintain safe work environment.
12. *Statistical monitoring*: It comprises the review at regular intervals of collected data on the health and environmental exposure of occupational group.
13. *Research*: It can provide a better understanding of the industrial health problems. There are two kinds of research—pure research and research for improvement of or in connection with a manufacturing product.

Statutory/Legislation Measures

To comply (in India) some main code/act like:

1. Occupational Safety, Health and Working Condition (OSH and WC) Code, 2020.
2. The ESI Act, 1948.
3. The Workmen's Compensation Act, 1923.

Administrative Measures

Examples:

Acclimatization: It is done to the workers who are going to absorb in heat prone areas.

Change of Job: Shifting of the workers from noisy area to non-noisy area who are suffering from NITTS or initial stage of noise induced hearing loss (NIHL).

NOTIFIABLE OCCUPATIONAL DISEASES

Notifiable Occupational Diseases under Indian Factories Act, 1948

National Laws and Regulations require the notification of some cases and suspected cases of occupational disease and these occupational diseases are called notifiable occupational diseases. These diseases are recognized internationally for the purpose of workmen's compensation. The main purpose of notification in industry is to initiate measure for prevention and protection and ensuring their effective application and to investigate the working conditions and other circumstances, which have caused or suspected to have caused occupational diseases.

Section 89, Notice of Certain Diseases

1. Where any worker in a factory contracts any disease specified in the [third] schedule the manager of the factory shall send notice thereof to such authorities, and in such form and within such time, as may be prescribed.
2. If any medical practitioner attends on a person, who is or has been employed in a factory, and who is, or is believed by the medical practitioner to be suffering from any disease specified in the third schedule, the medical practitioner shall without delay send a report in writing to the office of the chief inspector stating:
   a. The name and full postal address of the patient.
   b. The disease from which he believes the patient to be suffering.
   c. The name and address of the factory in which the patient is, or was last, employed.
3. Where the report under sub-section (2) is confirmed to the satisfaction of the chief inspector, by the certificate of the certifying surgeon or otherwise, that the person is suffering from a disease specified in the third schedule, he shall pay to the medical practitioner such fee as may be prescribed, and the fee so paid shall be recoverable as an arrears of land revenue from the occupier of the factory in which the person contracted the diseases.
4. If any medical practitioner fails to comply with the provisions of sub-section (2), he shall be punishable with fine which may extend to [Rs. 1000].
5. The Central Government may, by notification in the official gazette, add to or alter the third schedule and any such addition or alteration shall have effect as if it had been made by this act.

Section 90, Power to Direct Inquiry into Cases of Accident or Diseases

1. The State Government may, if it considers it expedient so to do, appoint a competent person to inquire into the cases of any accident occurring in a factory or into any case where a disease specified in the third schedule has been, or is suspected to have been, contracted in a factory, and may also appoint one or more persons possessing legal or special knowledge to act as assessors in such inquiry.
2. The person appointed to hold an inquiry under this section shall have all the powers of a Civil Court under the Code of Civil Procedure, 1908 (V of 1908), for the purposes of enforcing the attendance of witnesses and compelling the production of documents and material objects and may also, so far may be necessary for the purposes of the inquiry, exercise any of the powers of an Inspector under this Act; and every person required by the person making the inquiry to furnish any information shall be deemed to be legally bound so to do within the meaning of section 176 of the Indian Penal Code (XLV of 1960).
3. The person holding an inquiry under this section shall make a report to the State Government stating the cause of the accident or as the case may be, disease, and any attendant circumstances, and adding any observations which he or any of the assessors may think fit to make.
4. The State Government may, if it thinks fit, cause to be published any report made under this section or any extracts there from.
5. The State Government may make rules for regulating the procedure at inquiries under this section.

List of Notifiable Occupational Diseases as per the Factories Act, 1948: It is also recommended in Scheduled III of "The Occupational Safety, Health and Working Condition Code, 2020":

1. Lead poisoning including poisoning by any preparation or compound of lead or their sequelae.
2. Lead tetraethyl poisoning.
3. Phosphorus poisoning or its sequelae.
4. Mercury poisoning or its sequelae.
5. Manganese poisoning or its sequelae.
6. Arsenic poisoning or its sequelae.
7. Poisoning by nitrous fumes.
8. Carbon bisulfide poisoning.
9. Benzene poisoning, including poisoning by any of its homologues, their nitro or amino derivatives or its sequelae.
10. Chrome ulceration or its sequelae.
11. Anthrax.
12. Silicosis.
13. Poisoning by halogens or halogen derivatives of the hydrocarbons, of the aliphatic series.
14. Pathological manifestation due to:
    a. Radium and other radioactive substances.
    b. X-ray.
15. Primary epitheliomatous cancer of the skin.
16. Toxic anemia.
17. Toxic jaundice due to poisonous substances.
18. Oil acne or dermatitis due to mineral oils and compounds containing mineral oil base.
19. Byssinosis
20. Asbestosis.
21. Occupational or contact dermatitis caused by direct contact with chemical and paints. These are of types, i.e. primary irritant and allergic sensitizers.
22. Noise induced hearing loss (exposure to high noise levels).
23. Beryllium poisoning.
24. Carbon monoxide.
25. Coal miners' pneumoconiosis.
26. Phosgene poisoning.
27. Occupational cancer.
28. Isocyanates poisoning.
29. Toxic nephritis.

COMPENSATION FOR OCCUPATIONAL DISEASES

The Workmen's Compensation Act (renamed as Employees Compensation Act, 1923) is the first piece of legislation towards social security. It deals with compensation for workers who are injured in the course of duty. The scheme of the Workmen's Compensation Act is not to compensate the worker in lieu of wages. The general principle is that a worker who suffers an injury in the course of his employment, which results in a disablement, should be entitled to compensation and in the case of a fatal injury his dependants should be compensated. Under the Workmen's Compensation Act it is the employer who is responsible to pay compensation (as opposed to the Employees State Insurance, establishments to which the Employees' State Insurance Act applies to the liability to pay compensation is on the ESI Corporation). The meaning of compensation in this Act is limited to compensation granted under the Act for employment injuries sustained during the course of work.

As per Section 3 of the Act, the employer is liable to pay compensation if the worker is injured by accident that:

1. Arises out of (i.e. while engaged in work)
2. In the course of his employment (i.e. during workhours)
3. Such an injury results in disablement of the worker.

If three conditions are met, the employer of an establishment covered by the Act is bound to pay compensation. While the second condition, i.e. during work hours is easy to prove, the first condition (i.e. the accident occurred while engaged in work) has been difficult to establish in certain cases.

Compensation is not payable by the employer in the following circumstances:

1. Where the disablement does not last for >3 days.
2. Where the disablement has arisen out of the following:
   a. Drugs or drink
   b. Disobedience
   c. Disregard for the safety measures prescribed.

An 'occupational disease' while in service, is a disease that inflicts workers in that particular occupation in which s/he was employed in and resulting from exposure to a hazardous working atmosphere, particular to that employment. If a worker contracts such a disease, then the employer is liable to pay compensation, provided that the worker was employed by him for a continuous period of 6 months. An occupational disease that is contracted in the course of employment will fall within the meaning of an 'accident' for the purposes of this Act. In the case of such a disease being contracted, the employer will be liable to pay compensation to the affected worker. The occupational diseases for which compensation is payable are specified in a list attached to the Act-specifically, Part A of Schedule III.

The compensation to be paid (according to the Chapter 3 of the Act) by the employer for injuries caused depends on extent of the disablement suffered by the worker; more severe disablements naturally receive higher compensation. This has been categorized as follows:

Compensation payable in case of:

1. Death
2. Disablement:
   a. Permanent total disablement.
   b. Permanent partial disablement.
   c. Temporary disablement.
      i. Temporary total disablement.
      ii. Temporary partial disablement.

In addition, the guiding principle is the higher the age of the injured worker, the lower the compensation.

S. no.	Occupational Disease	Employment
Part A		
1.	Infectious and parasitic diseases contracted in an occupation where there is a particular risk of contamination.	(a) All work involving exposure to health or laboratory work (b) All work involving exposure to veterinary work (c) Work relating to handling animals, animal carcasses, part of such carcasses, or merchandise which may have been contaminated by animals or animal carcasses (d) Other work carrying a particular risk of contamination
2.	Diseases caused by work in compressed air	All work involving exposure to the risk concerned
3.	Diseases caused by lead or its toxic compounds	All work involving exposure to the risk concerned
4.	Poisoning by nitrous fumes	All work involving exposure to the risk concerned
5.	Poisoning by organophosphorus compounds	All work involving exposure to compounds the risk concerned
Part B		
1.	Diseases caused by phosphorus or its toxic compounds	All work involving exposure to the risk concerned
2.	Diseases caused by mercury or its toxic compounds	All work involving exposure to the risk concerned
3.	Diseases caused by benzene or its toxic homologues	All work involving exposure to the risk concerned
4.	Diseases caused by nitro and amino toxic derivates of benzene or its homologues	All work involving exposure to the risk concerned
5.	Diseases caused by chromium or its toxic compounds	All work involving exposure to the risk concerned
6.	Diseases caused by arsenic or its toxic compounds	All work involving exposure to the risk concerned
7.	Diseases caused by radioactive substances and ionising radiations	All work involving exposure to the action of radioactive substances or ionising radiations
8.	Primary epitheliomatous cancer of the skin the skin caused by tar, pitch, bitumen, mineral oil, anthracene, or the compounds, products or residues of these substances	All work involving exposure to the risk concerned
9.	Diseases caused by the toxic halogen derivatives of hydrocarbons (of the aliphatic and aromatic series)	All work involving exposure to the risk concerned
10.	Diseases caused by carbon disulfide	All work involving exposure to the risk concerned
11.	Occupational cataract due to infrared radiations	All work involving exposure to the risk concerned
12.	Diseases caused by manganese or its toxic compounds	All work involving exposure to the risk concerned
13.	Skin diseases caused by physical chemical or biological agents not included in other items	All work involving exposure to the risk concerned
14.	Hearing impairment caused by noise	All work involving exposure to the risk concerned

Table: List of occupational diseases as per Schedule III

(Contd.)

S. no.	Occupational Disease	Employment
15.	Poisoning by dinitrophenol or a homologue or by substituted dinitrophenol or by the salts of such substances	All work involving exposure to the risk concerned
16.	Disease caused by beryllium or its toxic compounds	All work involving exposure to the risk concerned
17.	Diseases caused by cadmium or its toxic compounds	All work involving exposure to the risk concerned
18.	Occupational asthma caused by recognised sensitising agents inherent in the work process	All work involving exposure to the risk concerned
19.	Diseases caused by fluorine or its toxic compounds	All work involving exposure to the risk concerned
20.	Diseases caused by nitorglycerine or other nitroacid esters	All work involving exposure to the risk concerned
21.	Diseases caused by alcohols and ketones	All work involving exposure to the risk concerned
22.	Diseases caused by asphyxiants: carbon monoxide, and its toxic derivates, hydrogen sulfide	All work involving exposure to the risk concerned
23.	Lung cancer and mesotheliomas caused by asbestos	All work involving exposure to the risk concerned
24.	Primary neoplasm of the epithelial lining of the urinary bladder or the kidney or the ureter	All work involving exposure to the risk concerned
25.	Snow blindness in snow bound areas	All work involving exposure to the risk concerned
26.	Disease due to effect of heat in extreme hot climate	All work involving exposure to the risk concerned
27.	Disease due to effect of cold in extreme cold climate	All work involving exposure to the risk concerned
Part C		
1.	Pneumoconioses caused by sclerogenic mineral dust (silicosis, anthracosilicosis, asbestosis) and silicotuberculosis provided that silicosis is an essential factor in causing the resultant incapacity or death	All work involving exposure to the risk concerned
2.	Bagassosis	All work involving exposure to the risk concerned
3.	Bronchopulmonary diseases caused by cotton, flax hemp and sisal dust (byssinosis)	All work involving exposure to the risk concerned
4.	Extrinsic allergic alveolitis caused by the inhalation of organic dusts	All work involving exposure to the risk concerned
5.	Bronchopulmonary diseases caused by hard metals	All work involving exposure to the risk concerned
6.	Acute pulmonary edema of high altitude	All work involving exposure to the risk concerned

EVALUATION OF INJURIES

Annexure 3

Schedule I

List of injuries deemed to result in permanent total disablement	
S. no. Description of injury percentage of loss of earning capacity	
Part I	
1. Loss of both hands or amputation at higher sites	100
2. Loss of hand and a foot	100
3. Double amputation through leg or thigh, or amputation through leg or thigh on one side and loss of others foot	100
4. Loss of sight to such an extent as to render the claimant unable to perform any work for which eyesight is essential	100
5. Very severe facial disfigurement	100
6. Absolute deafness	100
Part II	
1. Amputation through shoulder joint	90
2. Amputation below shoulder with stump <20.32 cm from tip of acromion	80
3. Amputation from 20.32 cm from tip of acromion to <11.43 cm below tip of olecranon	70
4. Loss of hand or of the thumb and four fingers of one hand or amputation from 11.43 cm below tip of olecranon	60
5. Loss of thumb	30
6. Loss of thumb and its metacarpal bone	40
7. Loss of four fingers of one hand	50
8. Loss of three fingers of one hand	30
9. Loss of two fingers of one hand	20
10. Loss of terminal phalanx of thumb	20
10A. Guillotine amputation of tip of thumb without loss of bone	10
Amputation cases–lower limbs	
11. Amputation of both feet resulting in end-bearing stumps	90
12. Amputation through both feet proximal to the metatarsophalangeal joint	80
13. Loss of all toes of both feet through metatarsophalangeal joint	40
14. Loss of all toes of both feet proximal to the proximal interphalangeal joint	30
15. Loss of all toes of both feet distal to the proximal interphalangeal joint	20
16. Amputation at hip	90
17. Amputation below hip with stump not exceeding 12.70 cm in length measured from tip of greater trochanter	80
18. Amputation below hip with stump exceeding 12.70 cm in length measured from tip of great trochanter but not beyond middle thigh	70
19. Amputation below middle thigh to 8.89 cm below knee	60
20. Amputation below knee with stump exceeding 8.89 cm but not exceeding 12.70 cm	50
21. Amputation below knee with stump exceeding 12.70 cm	50
22. Amputation of one foot resulting in end-bearing	50
23. Amputation through one foot proximal to the metatarsophalangeal joint	50
24. Loss of all toe of one foot through the metatarsophalangeal joint	20

(Contd.)

S. no.	Description of injury percentage of loss of earning capacity	
	Other injuries	
25.	Loss of one eye, without complications, the other being normal	40
26.	Loss of vision of one eye, without complications or disfigurement of eyeball, the other being normal	30
26A.	Loss of partial vision of one eye	10
	Fingers of right or left hand index finger	
27.	Whole	14
28.	Two phalanges	11
29.	One phalanx	9
30.	Guillotine amputation of tip without loss of bone	5
	Middle finger	
31.	Whole	12
32.	Two phalanges	9
33.	One phalanx	7
34.	Guillotine amputation of tip without loss of bone	4
	Ring or little finger	
35.	Whole	7
36.	Two phalanges	6
37.	One phalanx	5
38.	Guillotine amputation of tip without loss of bone	2
	Toes of right or left foot	
	Great toe	
39.	Through metatarsophalangeal joint	14
40.	Part, with some loss of bone	3
	Any other toe	
41.	Through metatarsophalangeal joint	3
42.	Part, with some loss of bone	1
	Two toes of one foot, excluding great toe	
43.	Through metatarsophalangeal joint	5
44.	Part, with some loss of bone	2
	Three toes of one foot, excluding great toe	
45.	Through metatarso-phalangeal joint	6
46.	Part, with some loss of bone	3
	Four toes of one foot, excluding great toe	
47.	Through metatarsophalangeal joint	9
48.	Part, with some loss of bone	3

Note: Complete and permanent loss of the use of any limb or member referred to in this Schedule shall be deemed to be equivalent to be loss of that limb or member.

Examples

Sample of the evaluation of an injury: Loss of earning capacity assessment in case of head injury in an Oil Industry in India

Loss of earning capacity	*Criteria*
40%	Head injury without EEG abnormality
50%	Head injury with EEG abnormality but without epileptic fit
60%	(a) Head injury with EEG abnormality and epileptic fit (b) Head injury with brain scarring and EEG abnormality
80%	Head injury with mental and physical disability without complete recovery
100%	Head Injury followed by invalidity

Hearing impairment evaluation:

Procedure: The following procedure is used to convert hearing threshold levels into percentages of hearing impairment, according to the 1979 AAOO (American Academy of Ophthalmology and Otolaryngology) formula:

1. The average of the hearing threshold level at 500, 1000, 2000 and 3000 Hz is calculated for each year.
2. The percent impairment for each ear is calculated by 1.5% the amount by which the aforementioned average hearing threshold level exceeds 25 dB (low fence). A maximum of 100% is reached at 92% dB (high fence).
3. The binaural impairment assessment should then be calculated by multiplying the smaller percentage (better ear) by 5, adding this figure to the larger percentage (poorer) and dividing the total by 6.

Sample of hearing loss calculation: Following are examples of the calculation of hearing loss:

Mild to marked bilateral hearing loss				
Ear	*500 Hz*	*1000 Hz*	*2000 Hz*	*3000 Hz*
Right	15	25	45	55
Left	40	50	60	70

1. Calculation of average hearing threshold level:
   Right ear = (15 + 25 + 45 + 55)/4 = 35 dB = 15% loss
   Left ear = (40 + 50 + 60 + 70)/4 = 55 dB = 45% loss
2. Calculation of the hearing handicapped:
   Smaller number (better ear): 15% × 5 = 75%
   Larger number (poorer ear) = 45%
   Total = (75 + 45)/6 = 20%

Therefore, a person with hearing threshold levels shown in this diagram would have a 20% hearing handicapped.

MEDICAL SERVICE IN AN INDUSTRIAL ESTABLISHMENT AND ITS FUNCTIONS

Medical service in an industrial establishment means a service established in or near a place of employment for the purpose of:

1. Protecting the workers against any health hazard which may arise out of their work or the conditions in which it is carried.
2. Contribution towards the workers' physical and mental adjustment.
3. Contribution to the establishment and maintenance of the highest possible degree of physical, mental and social well-being of the workers.
4. Facilitate the complete treatment of the workers and their families.

Medical Service Organization in Industry may be of following types: It depends on the circumstances and the applicable standard, set up of Medical Service Organization. They are:

1. Possible:
   a. Should eighter be organized by the undertaking themselves or be attached to an outside body.
   b. Should be organized as a:
      i. Separate service within a single undertaking
      ii. Service common to a number of undertakings.
2. Immediately not possible: Where medical services cannot immediately be set up for the undertaking, such service should be established in first instance:
   i. For undertaking where the health risks appear greatest
   ii. For undertaking where the workers are exposed to special health hazards.
3. Not at all possible: The organizations where the medical service is not practicable, they should make arrangement with a physician or a local medical service for:
   i. Administering emergency treatment
   ii. Carrying out medical examination
   iii. Exercising surveillance over hygiene conditions.

Functions of Medical Services in Industry

1. Surveillance of all factors which may affect the health of the workers.
2. Job analysis in the light of hygienic, physiological and psychological considerations.
3. Supervision of personal protective equipment and its use.
4. Supervision of the welfare of the workers.
5. Medical examinations of the workers.
6. Surveillance of the adaptation of jobs to workers, mainly the handicapped workers.
7. Rehabilitation of disabled workers.
8. Placement of workers in a safe condition from hazardous condition.
9. Advice to individual worker at their request regarding any disorder in the course of work.
10. Immediate treatment of medical and surgical emergencies.
11. Training to the first-aid personnel.
12. Health education.
13. Compilation and periodic review of statistics.
14. To maintain relation with internal and external services and bodies dealing with health, safety, retraining, rehabilitation and welfare of workers.

15. Organized medical board.
16. Notification.
17. Maintain confidential personal medical file.
18. Referred the case to the referral center for appropriate treatment.
19. To conduct health exhibition.
20. Health care activities for workers and their families.
21. Disaster management activities.
22. Take part in the safety committee.
23. Work place health monitoring.
24. To provide health facility to the surrounding populations as a part of corporate-social responsibility.
25. To maintain first-aid boxes in the industry.
26. Screening for substances of abuse and combating abuses.
27. Development of health policy and programme.
28. To conduct biological monitoring and investigations.
29. To conduct work environment monitoring.
30. Research.

OCCUPATIONAL HEALTH SERVICES AND ITS ACTIVITIES

Occupational Health Services (OSH) are human-service organizations in modern society which have been explicitly designed to manage and promote the safety, health and welfare of citizens at work. The role of OHS should be essentially preventive. They will evaluate their preventive program, discover occupational hazards, and recommend the suitable placement of workers.

Principles of OHS

a. *Preventive*: Preventing occupational health hazards at work, like inoculations (vaccination), enclosure of hazardous process, machine guard, etc.
b. *Health promotion*: Promoting physical, mental and social well-being of workers like canteen facility, industrial training, etc.
c. *Protective*: Protecting workers' health against hazards at work, like use of PPE.
d. *Adaptation*: Adopting work and work environment to the capabilities of the workers, like acclimatization.
e. *Cure and rehabilitation*: Curing and rehabilitating occupational accidental injuries, occupational and work-related diseases, like early diagnosis and treatment, change of job, etc.
f. *Primary health care*: To provide primary health care to the workers and their families like to provide all facilities of primary health center.

Occupational Health Professionals

They include:

- Occupational health physicians and nurses
- Physiotherapists and ergonomists
- Occupational hygienists
- Safety engineers
- Occupational psychologists
- Managers of OHS units or organizations.

Activities of OHS

- Survey of factors which affect occupational health
- Job analysis
- Medical examinations of the workers
- Supervision of the welfare of the workers
- Supervision of personal protective equipment
- Adaptation of job for the workers
- Rehabilitation of disable workers
- Recommendation for the placement of workers in suitable job
- Notification of the notifiable occupational diseases
- Maintenance of confidential personal medical files
- Training on occupational health
- Health education
- To conduct medical board
- Referred the cases to referral center
- Maintained relation with external and internal services dealing with health, safety, hygiene, training, rehabilitation and welfare of workers
- Early diagnosis and treatment
- To provide ergonomic intervention technique
- Compilation and periodic review of statistics
- Research.

Action Plan of OHS

- Strengthening of international and national policies for health at work and developing the necessary policy tools
- Development of healthy work environment
- Development of healthy work practices and promotion of health at work
- Strengthening of occupational health care system
- Establishment of appropriate support services for occupational health
- Development of occupational health standards based on scientific risk assessment
- Development of human resources for occupational health
- Establishment of registration and data system, development of information services for experts, effective transmission of data and raising of public awareness through public information
- Strengthening of research
- Development of collaboration on occupational health with other organizations.

OCCUPATIONAL HEALTH HAZARDS IN HOSPITAL

Human health service sectors, like all complex employment settings or industries have the usual variety of routine employee hazards along with special risks unique for these environments. Because of the progression of the medical technology and the emergence of new and re-emergence of old diseases, human health service sectors like hospitals have not become safer places for work.

1. **Biological hazards:** Infectious disease continues to represent the most serious and life-threatening to the workers working in the health service sectors. Not only do hospital personnel contract disease through exposure to infected patients, they actually can transmit disease, since they are dealing with immunocompromised individuals. Hospital acquired infection is known as 'nosocomial infection' and usually resistant to normal treatment. Followings are some biological hazards (infective) of healthcare workers and risk of transmission to patients:
    a. *Hepatitis B*: Acute icteric hepatitis, sometimes fulminant, can occur 3–6 months after occupational exposure to the virus in non-immune workers. Acutely or chronically infected healthcare workers who undertake exposure-prone procedures can transmit hepatitis B infection to their patients.
    b. *Hepatitis C (HCV)*: It is now known that HCV is the cause of large proportion of cases of what was formerly called 'non-A, non-B hepatitis'. Acute or and even fulminant hepatitis can occur after occupational transmission of HCV.
    c. *Human immunodeficiency virus (HIV)*: A seroconversion illness typically occurs about 4–6 weeks after the exposure. The potential for HIV-infected healthcare workers to transmit to patients during exposure-prone procedures is a cause of great concern, given the very serious consequences of such an occurrence.
    d. *Viral hemorrhagic fevers*: It is caused by a range of viruses and they are severe and life-threatening diseases. The infections are transmitted to humans by mosquito bite (yellow fever, dengue), tick bite (hemorrhagic fever) or through contact with virus excreted by infected rodents or others animal reservoir (Lassa virus).
    e. *SARS coronavirus*: Very recently a pandemic outbreak started in the 1st week of December, 2019 and this coronavirus outbreak continued several months killing thousands of people worldwide. This pandemic infectious disease is spreading all over the world. World Health Organization (WHO) has given the official name of this Novel Coronavirus as COVID-19.
    f. *Varicella zoster.*
    g. *Cytomegalovirus.*
    h. *Measles, mumps and rubella.*
    i. *Tuberculosis.*
    j. *Scabies.*
    k. *Staphylococcal infection.*
2. **Chemical hazards:**
    a. *Waste anesthetic gases*: A variety of adverse health effects that have been attributed to exposure to waste anesthetic gases include cancer, somatic complaints like headache and nausea, stillbirth, low birth weight, spontaneous abortion, congenital anomalies, and premature death.
    b. *Chemotherapeutic agents*: The chemotherapeutic agents have well-known toxic effects like myelosuppression, immunosuppression, and specific organ toxicity. The obvious direct consequence is a concern for health care workers who utilize these agents on a regular basis.

c. *Other chemical agents*: A myriad of agents has been demonstrated to show toxic effects in health care workers, including latex surgical gloves (which can produce both cutaneous and systemic hypersensitivity reactions), glutaraldehyde (it is used as a tissue fixative and as a cold sterilizing agent like ethylene oxide for heat sensitive medical equipment, it is volatile, and irritant skin and mucous membrane symptoms are common, therefore protective gloves should be used), psyllium, and ribavirin aerosol. Biomaterials (methyl methacrylate monomer and chromium-cobalt-molybdenum particles) have been reported to produce occupational health hazards including pneumoconiosis in dentistry. Methyl methacrylate monomer is usually used by the orthopedic surgeons as bone cement for implantation of prosthetics or for fixation in the placement of stabilizing screws or devices. Formaldehyde is also produced chemical health hazard in hospital.

3. **Mechanical hazards (traumatic injury):** Hospital workers are susceptible to back injury, especially to the direct patient caregivers. One risk factor is the caregiver-patient size mismatch when a small nurse tries to reposition a large patient in bed. Needle pricks to the health workers mainly to the doctors and nurses are a major cause of spreading the infectious diseases like HIV and hepatitis-B.
4. **Physical hazards:** Ionizing radiation is one of the most well recognized hazards in the hospital environment. Each hospital must have safety officers who are responsible for the areas of diagnostic radiology, nuclear medicine with its multiple isotopes, and radiotherapy units. Personal monitoring (film badge) is used to check the adequacy of the radiation protection programme for the radiology employees. Pregnant lady is not allowed to be exposed to ionizing radiation, e.g. X-ray. X-ray technician should have to take adequate protection or personal protective equipment like lead coated apron or protected enclosure.
5. **Psychosocial hazards:** Work stress in most production-oriented organization is high but the stress for health care workers is compounded by the knowledge that mistake can cause significant harm to patients. Life and death decisions made almost instantly are not uncommon, and long hours with inadequate staffing compound the problem. House staff suffers extreme stress compounded by very long duty hours. Employee assistance programmes have proven to be useful in hospital setting, as they are in other environments.

Preventive and Control Measures

A. General measures:

i. Personal hygiene and environmental sanitation: Keep it at high level in the hospital of any kind, is a mandatory requirement towards control of hospital infection.

ii. Efficient housekeeping including clean supply of bed-liner, patients' dress, proper bed arrangement, frequent moping, periodic washing of ward floor.

iii. Provision of auxiliary facilities like:

a. Central Sterile Supply Department (CSSD)

b. Mechanized laundry

c. Hygienic kitchen and food supply system

d. Prompt and coordinated system of waste management, and good housekeeping.

B. Special control:

i. Air conditioning through fresh filtered air
ii. Washing and disinfection of hospital ward in periodic interval
iii. Periodical biological test of the swab
iv. Plenty of water supply in the hospital
v. Use of PPE like lead-coated apron for X-ray technician and use of protective gloves, masks, etc.

Principles of waste disposal in hospitals: Proper management of medical waste comprises collection, packaging, storage, transport, treatment, recycling, and disposal within the medical institution (station, ambulance, laboratory) up to the final disposal (recycling, thermal treatment, landfill).

ACTION PROGRAM FOR WORK RELATED DISEASES AT NATIONAL LEVELS

Hearing Conservation Program

Noise is not only a health problem but also a legal one as noise induced hearing loss (NIHL) in industrial workers due to industrial noise is compensable as per the Workman's Compensation Act. The compensation claims may amount to huge sums affecting the economy of the industries. Hence to safeguard workers from noise as well as to reduce compensation claims, 'Hearing Conservation Program' plays a vital role. The successful program must include the coordination and integration of four phases:

1. Physical evaluation of the noise exposure (noise measurement) and noise reduction.
2. Control of noise exposure (provision of personal ear protection).
3. Medical evaluation of hearing of exposed personnel (audiometric test).
4. Information and education.

Physical Evaluation of the Noise Exposure (Noise Measurement)

The relationship of hearing loss to noise exposure: With the development of accurate methods of measuring both the sound stimulus and the hearing level, more precise determination of relationship between hearing loss and noise exposure has become possible.

Noise reduction: Noise reduction can be helped by the enclosure of noisy machines, the use of mufflers, damping, silencers, anti-vibration mountings, the treatment of reflective surfaces with absorbing materials, the limitation of the use of noisy equipment to times when it is actually required, and the distancing the workers from the areas of maximum noise.

Control of noise exposure (provision of personal ear protection): Ear protection provides a system of attenuation of the incoming sound and thus minimizes the sound arriving at the tympanic membrane. Hearing protective devices is considered the last option for controlling noise exposure. These are usually used during the time it takes to implement engineering or administrative controls, or when such controls are not feasible. Unless great care is taken in establishing a hearing conservation program, workers will often receive very little benefit from hearing protective devices. The best hearing protector, when fitted correctly, is one that is accepted by the worker and worn properly. If the worker exposure is above 85 dBA (8-hour TWA), hearing protection must be made available, along with the other requirements in the hearing conservation program. Various types of protectors are available. Plants having hearing conservation program generally assign their medical departments the task of fitting employees with ear plugs, earmuffs and hearing protective helmets.

Noise reduction ratings: When OSHA promulgated its Hearing Conservation Amendment in 1983, it incorporated the EPA labeling requirements for hearing protectors (40 CFR 211), which required manufacturers to identify the noise reduction capability of all hearing protectors on the hearing protector package. This measure is referred to as the noise reduction rating (NRR). It is a laboratory-derived numerical estimate of the attenuation achieved by the protector. It became evident that the amount of protection users was receiving in the workplace with the prescribed hearing protectors did not correlate with the attenuation indicated by the NRR. OSHA acknowledged that in most cases, this number overstated the protection afforded to workers and required the application for certain circumstances of a safety factor of 50# to the NRR, above and beyond the 7 dB subtraction called for when using A-weighted measurements, e.g. consider a worker who is exposed to 98 dBA for 8 hours and whose hearing protectors have an NRR of 25 dB. We can estimate the worker's resultant exposure using the 50# safety factor. The worker's resultant exposure is 89 dBA in this case.

The 50# safety factor adjusts labeled NRR values for workplace conditions and is used when considering whether engineering controls are to be implemented.

Estimated dBA exposure = 98 dBA – [(25 – 7) × 50#] = 89 dBA

However, when assessing the adequacy of the hearing protection for hearing conservation (HC) purposes, CSHOs should only subtract 7 dB from the NRR.

Exposure for PPE/HC enforcement = 98 dBA – (25 – 7) = 80 dBA

Single/double hearing protection: Dual hearing protection involves wearing two forms of hearing protection simultaneously (e.g. earplugs and ear muffs). The noise exposure for workers wearing dual protection may be estimated by the following method: Determine the hearing protector with the higher rated NRR (NRRh) and subtract 7 dB if using A-weighted sound level data. Add 5 dB to this field-adjusted NRR to account for the use of the second hearing protector. Subtract the remainder from the TWA. It is important to note that using such double protection will add only 5 dB of attenuation.

Medical evaluation of hearing of exposed personnel (audiometric test): Industrial environments are seldom suitable for accurate tests of normal hearing, even though the medical facilities may be located in a relatively quit area. To determine the suitability of an area for audiometric testing, it is necessary to carry out environmental noise measurements during the noisiest anticipated conditions. From these studies, the degree of attenuation required to permit accurate threshold audiometry can be determined. In most instance, it will be cheaper and more satisfactory to purchase a prefabricated testing room (audiometry room/booth) having sufficient attenuation to permit accurate threshold measurements under the worst conditions.

Information and education: Workers at risk of occupational noise-induced hearing loss need to be educated about the harmful effects of noise and the importance of hearing conservation measures. They need to understand the important of wearing properly fitting and appropriate ear protections.

Vision Conservation Program

A well-recognized Vision Conservation Program for an industry has five components:

1. Screening the vision of the individual worker.
2. Determining the vision requirements of different jobs among the workers.
3. Detailed assessment of the hazards of the jobs with special reference to the eye and the general working environment.

4. Encouraging the wearing of basic eye protective equipment at all times by every worker who enters the area potentially hazardous to the eye.
5. Providing properly fitting and approved type of safety eye-wears against special type of hazardous operations.

Individual workers should be examined and vision status recorded: Both at the time of initial recruitment (pre-employment medical examination) and periodical medical examinations. A 'vision tester' or an 'Orthorator' is a very useful and compact instrument to screen acuity of vision (both distant and near), field of vision, muscle balance (in both the planes), binocular vision and color vision. The visual standards of each worker should be carefully matched with the vision requirements of jobs performed by them, e.g. crane operators and drivers.

MAJOR ACCIDENT HAZARDS CONTROL—MEDICAL PROVISION

It is the statutory requirement of the occupier of any hazardous industry to have an emergency medical preparedness plan. Preparedness and preventive measures are not same.

Preparedness: It covers all actions taken with a view to organizing and facilitating timely and effective rescue, relief and rehabilitation.

Prevention: It means the formulation and implementation of long-term policies and measures to mitigate the impact. A well established and functioning enterprise level occupational health service (OHS) scheme forms the basis of Major Accident Hazard Control Scheme.

Medical Organization for Emergencies

The most important factor in the relationship between the prognosis of victims and the interval of time elapsing between sustaining the injuries are the availability of medical care. This later period is called the "delay-time or reaction time or response time". The emergency medical responses aimed at in reducing the 'delay-time'. As a general rule a casualty is ought to be offered the treatment at the earliest possible time.

The medical organization for getting the proper responses in emergency (industrial major accidents) has mainly three components.

1. Organization at Site (On-site Emergency)

Medical organization at site is needed for the purpose of:

a. Early identification.
b. Elimination of human error risk factors due to physiological and pathological causes.
c. Planning and executing the rescue operation.
d. Effective first-aid management.
e. Training for minimizing the after effects of major accident.
f. Constitution of 'Trauma team' for rescue and first-aid operations.

Effectiveness of on-site medical organization depends on:

a. Capability of the personnel.
b. Availability of trauma team.
c. Plan of action to receive the victims.
d. Their codification.

e. Their first-aid treatment.
f. Transportation.

Function of Trauma Team

Appropriate emergency first-aid treatment at the earliest:

1. To reduce delay time or reaction time: quick removal of the casualties from disaster site.
2. Prevention of respiratory failure and administration of oxygen.
3. Control of bleeding.
4. Replacement of suitable fluid for loss of blood.
5. Treatment of shock.
6. Replacement of suitable painkillers.
7. Supportive treatment for cardiac, respirator and other systems.
8. Splinting and immobilization in case of fractures.
9. To keep the body warm with blankets and to protect open wounds with suitable sterile dressing.
10. Moral support to the injured.
11. Maintenance of medical records.
12. Dead body, if any, is to be identified and dealt in the appropriate manner.
13. Distribution to the injured to referral center.

Action Plan

1. Employees should be trained first aid and be available at short notice to take part in the rescue operation.
2. Periodical mock drill should be conducted so that each one knows his exact role and responsibility.
3. Liaison with nearby reference hospital.
4. All employees should have had their blood grouped and routine immunization carried out.
5. A mutual aid-scheme should be worked out in case of an industrial complex.
6. A system of 'Triage' is to be adopted to classified the victims into different groups depending upon the severity of the injury and urgency of transportation:
   a. Category I (Red tag): Highest priority.
   b. Category II (Blue tag): Highest priority.
   c. Category III (Yellow tag): Second priority.
   d. Category IV (Green tag): Lowest priority.
   e. Category X (Black tag): Least priority.

Triage System

The process of triage is used, to sort out patients into categories of priority for care and transport, based on the severity of injuries and medical emergencies. The sorting of patients begins as soon as trained personnel reach the site or sees the sick and injured persons.

Through careful triage, the patients can be placed into one of three categories: *Highest priority, second priority* and *lowest priority*.

Highest priority: Category I with red tag will get the highest priority from the medical point of view. The category I means: the victim is seriously injured, required immediate hospitalization in the referral center with life-supporting equipment during transportation. Category II with blue tag will get the same priority. The category II means the victim is seriously injured, required immediate hospitalization in the referral center without any life-supporting equipment during transportation. Examples of highest priority cases:

1. Respiratory arrest, airway obstruction, and severe breathing difficulties.
2. Cardiac arrest (remember that respiratory arrest is usually detected first).
3. Uncontrolled severe bleeding.
4. Severe head injuries.
5. Open chest wounds.
6. Open abdominal wounds.
7. Severe shock.
8. Burns involving the respiratory tract.
9. Severe medical problems (including heart attack cardiac stroke, heatstroke, poisoning and abnormal childbirth).
10. Unconsciousness.

Second priority: Category III with yellow tag will get the second priority. The category III means: victim is injured, required hospitalization in the referral center but not immediately.

1. Injuries to the spine (including cervical spine).
2. Moderate bleeding.
3. Conscious patients with head injuries.
4. Multiple fractures.

Lowest priority: Category IV with green tag will get lowest preference. The victim is injured required only first aid treatment and allows to go home. Category X with black tag will get least priority as the victim is dead or going to die.

1. Minor bleeding.
2. Minor fractures and minor soft tissue injuries.
3. Moderate and minor burns.
4. Obvious mortal wounds where survival is not expected.
5. Obvious death.

Transportation of Victims (Communication)

The transportation and allocation of victims to the hospitals need to be organized. The medical care rendered during transportation induces complications. There shall be two types of ambulances: one having life-supporting equipment and other without life-supporting equipment. Networking and round the clock readiness should be the essential feature of ambulance services. For this coordination between concerned agencies is necessary. Ambulance shall be manned by a full time driver-cum-mechanic and a helper trained in first aid, for the purposes of transportation of serious cases of accidents or sickness. The ambulance van shall not be used for any purpose other than the purpose stipulated herein and will normally be stationed at or near to the Occupational Health Center.

2. Organization in the Hospital (Off-site Emergency Plan)

Primary requirement for drawing plans for the hospitals to cope with emergencies arising out of major accidents is the identification of the victims, codification, distribution and early medical management should be there. The time period should be also so arranged that the initiation of each segment of the plan is made in the least possible time.

Crash team: A well-planed and optimum medical response helps the victims in a great way. The chances of survival and reducing the complication increase with this. The availability of Crash Team adds to the efficiency of such organization. The team consists of one Surgeon, one Anesthetist, one medical specialist, one or two theatre sisters, one casualty sister with other supporting paramedical staffs.

3. Medical Responses from Non-medical Personnel/Organizations

1. Police
2. Civil defence
3. Fire-brigade
4. Transport
5. NGO
6. Local administration.

OCCUPATIONAL HEALTH AUDIT AND SURVEY

Unlike hospital medicine, occupational health has always been closely associated with industry and therefore the efforts directed at improving the quality of occupational health service (OHS) has closely linked to the strategies already being used by industry to improve the quality of their own services and products.

Some occupational health departments have adopted the ISO-9000/BS-5750 approach and have incorporated elements of both medical and clinical audit into quality system. In India, the Bureau of Indian Standard (BIS) as per their clause 14489 has renamed the traditional safety audit as occupational safety and health audit and incorporated occupational health audit elements there.

Objectives of Occupational Health Audit

1. To determine the effectiveness and efficiency of an OHS organization as a whole.
2. To determine the need of change, e.g. in policy and in other planning and to evaluate any changes implemented.
3. To evaluate the contribution of the healthcare professionals and hence to help identify and plan education, training and other interventions.
4. To determine compliance with a standard, or with a service level agreement in terms of the structure of services, the quality of their process and/or the effectiveness of outcome.
5. To aid communication and find gaps in the evidence base for current practice, for setting the agenda for further research, evaluation and hence wider improvements in quality.

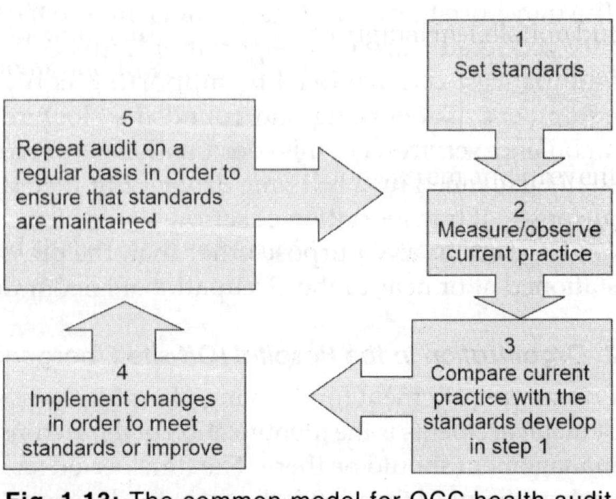

Fig. 1.13: The common model for OCC health audit

The most common approach to clinical audit on occupational health is based on Donabedian's structure, 'process and outcome' model (UK model) which uses techniques as the 'audit spiral' to help set standards, observe practice and compare current practice against the identified standard. In this model, changes can be introduced to ensure that the consistency of practice is maintained or to further improved the quality of practice. The standards set should be subjected to a rigorous process of continuous review, which takes account of new research and information generated from the audit process.

Elements of Occupational Health Audit

1. Occupational health administration.
2. Occupational health and hygiene program.
3. Occupational health service policy and procedures.
4. Health service resources facilities.
5. Health service program and activities.
6. Training program.
7. First-aid and medical program.
8. Records and forms.
9. Identification and assessment of occupational diseases.
10. Health surveillance and health monitoring.
11. Health and welfare measures.

Occupational Health Survey

Occupational health physicians are frequently asked to participate in work-site evaluation through occupational health survey. This evaluation may be performed to determine the work-relatedness of the single patient's symptoms, to investigate allegations of adverse health effects in a group of workers, to assist in the design of health and safety programs for a facility, or as a work-site 'follow-back' study of a sentinel health event. This workplace evaluation can range from brief walk-through surveys to more in-depth investigation including medical and environmental testing. The survey team usually consists of a medical officer and an industrial hygiene professional working together to perform a comprehensive evaluation of occupational hazards in a workplace.

Consultants conducting work-site evaluations should gather as much information as possible about the establishment before the site visit. Frequently this begins with a literature search centered around the materials and processes used. All work-site evaluation should begin with an opening conference led by the occupational health consultant. Attendees should include the plant manager, an individual responsible for plant health and safety, and at least one worker representative. The meeting should define the scope and nature of the investigation, address methodology of environmental and medical testing, and clarify concerns about trade secret and medical confidentiality issues. All attendees should be given the opportunity to ask questions or express concerns about the investigation process.

Once the opening conference is complete, the consultant team should devote some time to reviewing company health and safety records before actually beginning the walk-through. The reporting and recording systems can provide a good source of information about company injury and illness incidence rates. Logs from the company nurse, physician or first-aid center may give additional information about injury and illness that were not considered reportable. A material safety data sheet (MSDS) should be available for each toxic material used in the workplace; review of this information can identify many potential occupational hazards. Even a comprehensive set of MSDS may not reflect all chemical hazards in the workplace since reactive intermediates in the manufacturing process will not be reflected in this information. For example, the 1984 Bhopal disaster in India involved the release of methyl isocyanate, an intermediate in the production process of manufacturing the insecticide carbaryl.

Ideally, personal sampling data are available for a representative number of employees throughout the plant and have been correlated with appropriate medical or biological monitoring data. In reality, environmental monitoring data may be limited to area samples or to personal samples on a small number of workers. Individual work practices vary enough that two workers doing the same job in nearly identical settings may have quite different exposures. The use of personal protective equipment (PPE) may also modify individual exposures, although this is difficult to quantify. Workers may be using personal protective equipment without appropriate environmental data to demonstrate a need for it or to assist in appropriate selection. For example, many small firms require hearing protection in areas that are perceived as 'noisy', but have never conducted noise surveys. As a result, individuals who should be included in a hearing conservation program may not be, and individuals who work in noisy areas, especially those exposed to impact noise, may be inadequately protected. Similarly, the choice of appropriate respiratory protection also depends on adequate knowledge of the nature and level of air contaminants in the work environment.

When permitted, the occupational medical consultant should review any medical surveillance data collected through company programs. This may be difficult to access or look at systematically since a great percentage of occupational medical services are performed by outside clinics rather than in company facilities. Company may allow consulting physicians to review medical records that their employees have submitted in support of workers' compensation claims. If the consultation is being conducted in response to employee complaints, individual who have sought medical consultation relating to the occupational condition under investigation may voluntarily submit copies of their medical records for review.

In addition to the aforementioned medical and environmental information, the database of occupational health and safety consultations should be expanded to include information on company history, the formal statement of company goals, formal and informal organizational structure, labour-management relation, and regional economic trends.

The work-through evaluation itself is best accomplished by following the process from the entry of raw materials into the plant until the point where the finished product leaves the facility. This format should allow the consultant to see most job categories and departments and most routine job tasks. Maintenance activities and 'rework' of substandard product should be evaluated as well. Tasks that are performed infrequently or are not viewed as an integral part of the production process are often given little attention in company health and safety activities until they are associated with an injury or illness. The use of personal protective equipment in prescribed areas should be observed as well as employee hygiene practice such as eating, drinking, or smoking in potentially contaminated areas. The physicians should keep in mind that exposure may occur through inhalation, ingestion, dermal absorption, or a combination thereof, and should look for evidence of these as the walk-through is conducted.

During the walk-through, it is useful to ask employees about their work. Individual workers can often provide more insight into their specific job task than the plant representative present on the walk-through. Discussions regarding health problems should be brief, informal, and confidential. Initial question should be open-ended, rather than directed at specific symptoms or complaints. These can be followed with more specific questions about the nature, duration, timing and frequency of symptoms, as well as their association with work activities. It is also helpful to ask workers whether they know of any individuals who left employment with this company for health-related reasons.

If an industrial hygiene consultant is present, the walk-through survey may provide an opportunity for some limited environmental monitoring to help identify workplace contaminants and potential sources or exposure areas in the plant. Direct reading sampling equipment is available to assess airborne chemical contaminants, such as carbon monoxide, oxides of nitrogen, acid fumes and combusting hydrocarbons. Smoke tubes are a convenient means of observing airflow patterns relating to plant operations or ventilation systems; velocity meters can be used to obtain more exact information on plant ventilation.

The findings from the walk-through survey will suggest whether a potential occupational health hazard exists, and whether an in-depth medical or environmental survey, or both, is needed to characterize it. If environmental data demonstrates significant potential exposures, the industrial hygiene consultant may recommend either a thorough one-time survey or an ongoing monitoring program. Ongoing monitoring is particularly useful for exposures to agents whose health effects include long periods with asymptomatic changes and conditions that may benefit from early detection. Design of an in-depth medical survey should be based on findings from the walk-through and knowledge about the expected adverse health effects of substances used in the workplace.

When the work-site evaluation is complete, whether after the walk-through or following a more in-depth survey, a report should be issued that summarizes the findings of the investigation and makes appropriate recommendations for continuing health and safety activities within the establishment. For example, the industrial hygienist might recommend appropriate control technology or an ongoing environmental monitoring program. The occupational health physician may recommend, and help the company design, an ongoing medical surveillance program using appropriate screening tests to look for end-organ effects associated with the hazards encountered in the workplace. An understanding of the firm's organizational structure is critical to the consultants' ability to bring about change. The consultant must identify and have access to someone with enough authority to facilitate the acceptance and implementation of the final recommendations.

OCCUPATIONAL DISEASES RELATING TO CONSTRUCTION WORK, EMERGENCY MEDICAL TREATMENT OF INJURIES AND REHABILITATION AT CONSTRUCTION SITE

People might think that the active outdoor life in the construction industry would keep the workers fit and healthy. Quite the reverse is the true and the construction industry has a deservedly notorious reputation as being dirty, difficult and dangerous. Many people suffer fatal injuries on building sites every year. Many hundreds of thousands more people suffer serious injuries and ill health. Responsibilities for planning and coordination of health and safety are often unclear and compliance with health and safety law is generally poor. Informal contractual conditions in this sector make it difficult for workers to exercise their right and to push for more progressive and effective prevention initiatives based on workers participation, collective bargaining and training on skills, health and safety. The consequence of poor management standards in this sector is the deterioration of working and living conditions and an alarmingly high incidence of injuries.

Workers in construction industry are exposed to a wide range of hazardous substances and physical agents. Hazardous substances also have a serious impact on construction workers health. These may come in the form of liquids, gases, vapors, fumes or dusts. They are contained in a variety of commonly used products and materials in construction. The main exposure route is through inhalation, but substances such as solvents can also be absorbed through the skin. Very often, workers are not aware of what chemicals are contained in the products they use, and are not told about the health hazards and how to avoid them. The number one construction killer in any country is falling from height and this is principally due to the lack of proper edge protection in a variety of construction tasks. Height vertigo or height phobia is one of the important causes of fall from the height. Electrocution may also cause fatal and nonfatal injuries to the construction workers.

Most people are killed whilst carrying out perfectly routine work, where the hazards are well known. Deaths from these causes can and should be avoided by use of collective prevention measures. Lack of collective preventive measures is particularly dangerous when combined with work organization factors, i.e. management failures like poor housekeeping, chaotic working conditions, lack of planning and coordination, lack of training and supervision and intense productivity and time pressure.

Physical Hazards

Occupational deafness due to exposure of high noise level is very common in construction workers. Vibration syndrome mainly white fingers or Raynaud's phenomenon is common due to the use of vibrating pneumatic tools. Whole body vibration caused by operating heavy machinery and vehicles can cause damage to the spine. Extreme heat and cold, electrical injury, UV radiation from welding are some physical hazards in construction industry.

Chemical Hazards

Cement dust can cause serious respiratory problems over time, such as pneumoconiosis. Cement contains lots of chemicals, some of which cause skin problems like skin burn and contact dermatitis. Allergic dermatitis is caused by sensitivity to the chromium in cement and can be severe. Cement, fiberglass and wood preservatives can all cause irritant contact dermatitis, as well as mould oil in brick making. Cement burns are caused by wet cement trapped against the skin. Chromate and cobalt in cement, epoxy resin in special cements, softwoods and hardwoods, and rubber chemicals in boots and sealing strips are the main allergens.

Free silica dust can cause silicosis. This means irreversible scarring of the lungs, causing shortness of breath and premature death. Jobs such as stone masonry; concrete cutting or drilling; tunnelling and many demolition jobs can generate free silica.

Asbestos causes fatal diseases—asbestosis, mesothelioma and cancer of the lung. The use of asbestos in building and insulation materials has been widespread for many years. Millions of buildings all over the world contain asbestos, and workers carrying out maintenance, repairs, renovation or demolition work are often exposed without even being aware of it.

Wood dust causes respiratory system problems, irritation and allergy, asthma, rhinitis. Some types of wood dust and oils can cause nasal cancer, particularly certain hard woods. Fiber board and plywood contain glues and urea formaldehyde. Exposure to these chemicals may cause irritations.

Biological Hazards

Due to poor living and working condition of construction workers, many of them suffer from biological hazards like tuberculosis, cholera, parasitic diseases, dengue and malaria. Migration, including rural-urban migration, to seek work in large construction projects means being away from home and family for long periods. Therefore, the construction workers are at risk of HIV and AIDS (sexually transmitted diseases).

Mechanical Hazards

Back injuries may cause by manual handling of heavy loads, sometimes over long distances. For examples, bricks, cement blocks and cement bags with heavy load, confined spaces, awkward postures, heavy task and productivity demands, and long hours. Low back injuries, sciatica, hernias and slipped discs can put people out of the labor for ever. Other musculoskeletal disorders, injuries to muscles, nerves, tendons and joints are caused by physically demanding work. Risk factors include: uncomfortable postures, forceful and repetitive movements, awkward tools and sustained effort. Typical injuries include: Bursitis from kneeling, e.g. floor laying.

Psychosocial Hazards

Work stress of these workers may develop due to low socioeconomic condition, poor job security and high work stress.

Preventive Measures

Improvement can be made by substitution of hazardous materials for safer ones, by the introduction of safe working methods, by the use of appropriate PPE, through information, training and workers participation, access to occupational health services and health surveillance, providing social security and health schemes and strict implementation of law.

Caisson or Tunnelling Work

Caisson or tunnelling work is a part of civil engineering activity. Working at pressure becomes a requirement where excavation occurs beneath the level of the water table and where the ground is sufficiently porous to allow water to be forced into the tunnel or caisson as a result of the groundwater pressure. Hence, while it is possible to tunnel through solid impervious rock below water level without risk of flooding, tunnelling through softer water-permeable ground readily results in a water-filled tunnel with a risk of collapse of the tunnel apex or face. In this situation, to allow work to progress, the open end of the tunnel is closed off with a pressure tight structure and the tunnel is pressurized to a pressure adequate to prevent water ingress and stabilize the tunnel face. A pressure chamber or lock is built into the tunnel enclosure to allow workers to transfer from the surface to the pressurized environment without loss of pressure in the tunnel. This enables the tunnel construction to continue with work conducted in a dry environment.

Caissons are generally used for sinking bridge piers or structural foundation and furnish a means of removing mud and clay underwater so that bedrock may be reached upon which to place the foundation. A caisson is simply an inverted box that forms the bottom of the bridge pier. The edges of the box are bevelled so that they will cut into the clay or silt as weight is applied above. It is a large watertight chamber, open at the bottom, from which the water is kept out by air pressure and in which construction work may be carried out under water. Water is forced from the working compartment using compressed air, and the actual digging process can begin. Two shafts are provided which extend from the working chamber to the surface—one for removing mud and other excavated materials and one for the use of the working crew. A decompressed chamber is placed at the top where the working crew can decompress at the end of each shift.

Occasionally in caisson work, the physical layout makes it difficult to provide a large decompression chamber for the working crew in physical continuity with the shaft from the caisson below. In such cases, 'decanting' is used, wherein the workers decompressed very rapidly from the working pressure and then, within 5 minutes, move to a recompression chamber on an adjacent platform. However, decanting has the potential of producing a good deal of bubbling in the blood and tissues of the workers involved and, therefore, this process should be discouraged.

When the sand or muck becomes porous or the tunnel runs under a river or lake, there often is no practical way of keeping the water out except by putting considerable air pressure in the tunnel. To this purpose, an airtight bulkhead is erected across the tunnel so that pressure may be applied to the working face. Behind this bulkhead, a second bulkhead must be placed so that a decompression lock is created for the workers to enter and leave the work heading without having to drop the pressure on the heading itself.

Most tunnels are now constructed mechanically using a sophisticated tunnel boring machine (TBM) which lines the tunnel as it is constructed and hence the only human work requiring a pressurized environment is maintenance work conducted at the front face of the machine, such as blade or tool changing or technical or geological inspections. TBM requires short intense periods of compressed air interventions, sometimes at high pressures of 4–8 ATA. A shorter pressure exposure is now being adopted following recommendations from the medical advisers, especially where working pressure exceeded 2 ATA and this was eventually prescribed by HSE of UK in the 1996 regulations. Working pressure >3 ATA restrict shift duration. This has led to the need for the development and implementation of safer decompression techniques that give longer working time at higher pressure (>4 ATA) and with reduced risk of decompression sickness or dysbaric osteonecrosis. This means the application of diving technologies in the civil engineering context, which includes the use of mixed gas and saturated techniques, in addition to oxygen decompression. Tunnel workers may also require a gradual return to the surface pressure to prevent the onset of decompression illness. The decompression or ascent is conducted in a pressure lock so can be very accurately controlled.

Caisson and tunnel environments have other significant safety issues. They are enclosed (confine) spaces and require appropriate ventilation. Carbon dioxide retention may be a contributory factor in decompression illness. It is critical to ensure that the environment is not contaminated by toxic chemicals, particularly carbon monoxide (CO), and that all possible sources of ignition are controlled to avoid fire. Fire in a pressurized tunnel burns more intensely for a given flame size, spreads more vigorously and is harder to extinguish than atmospheric pressure and all of these effects are magnified by oxygen enrichment. So, the fire risk depends on both pressure and percentage of oxygen in the environment and remains a major safety consideration in compressed air work.

The followings are the conditions for compressed-air tunnel work:

1. Eat a well-balance diet.
2. Be temperate. Avoid excessive alcoholic beverages the night before or within 8 hours of going to shift.

3. Sleep at least 7 hours daily.
4. Take extra outer clothing into the tunnel when going on shift and during decompression to avoid chilling during that period.
5. Do not sit or rest in a cramped position during decompression.
6. Do not exercise during decompression. This does not mean you cannot move around to avoid sitting in one position.
7. Do not do hard exercise immediately after decompression.
8. Do not take a hot bath or shower within 6 hours of decompressing. A moderate warm bath or shower is permissible.
9. Do not go to sleep in a cramped position after decompression.
10. Do not allow yourself to become chilled within 6 hours after decompression.
11. Report at once to the physician incharge if you suspect you are suffering from "air pain" or decompression sickness. Do not give workers who are suffering from compressed-air illness any alcoholic drink.
12. If after decompressing, you develop 'niggles' or air pains that persists longer than a half hour, call the medical lock at once.
13. If you become ill away from the job site, communicate at once with the physician incharge.
14. Wear your identification bracelet so it will be known what to do with you in an emergency.
15. Stay within a 30-mile radius of the recompression facility for at least 1 hour after locking out.
16. Do not re-enter the man lock if suffering from 'air pains' or decompression sickness.
17. Do not fly in any aircraft for at least 12 hours after coming off shift.
18. Do not engage in any scuba diving (i.e. the simplest type of underwater breathing gear for the commercial diver, which is the self-contained rig consisting of bottles of air strapped to the driver's back and a demand regulator that supplies air to the diver via hose and mouthpiece at whatever pressure the person happens to be diving) at depths greater than 33 ft within 12 hours of coming off shift.
19. Do not engage in any scuba diving within 12 hours of going on shift.
20. Re-examination as per statutes.

The followings are the conditions that might disqualify a worker from compressed-air employment:

1. History of spontaneous pneumothorax.
2. History of ear surgery.
3. Active asthma.
4. Chronic embolism.
5. Addiction of narcotic or stimulant drugs.
6. Seizure disorders.
7. Pancreatitis.
8. Psychosis.
9. Gross obesity.
10. Advanced age.

Conditions that require close scrutiny:

1. Diabetes.
2. Hypertension.

3. History of thoracotomy.
4. History of fractures of the humerus or femur.
5. Migraine headaches.
6. History of taking systemic steroids.

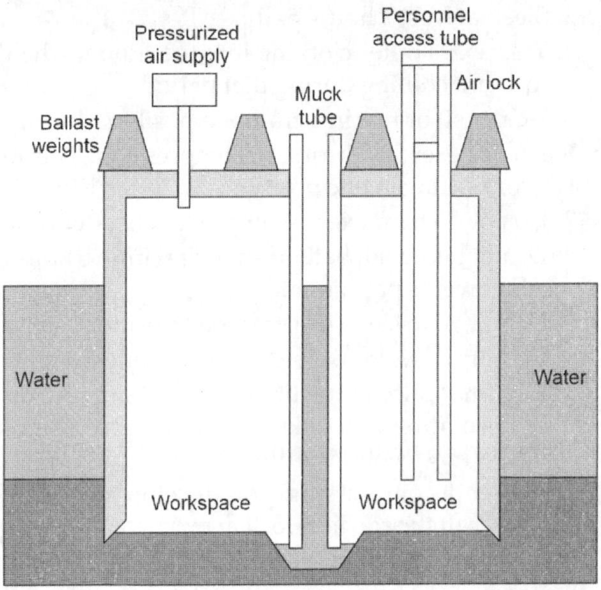

Fig. 1.14: Caisson engineering

Lifting of Loads in Industry

Lifting or carrying heavy loads, frequent bending or twisting, and heavy physical work may cause low back disorders. Lifting or carrying heavy loads has been linked to low back disorders in numerous publications. Epidemiological research has identified that the risk of injury increases when lifting loads from low heights, holding the load away from the body, or lifting while the torso is twisted or flexed. Biomechanical research supports these findings by demonstrating that loading of the spine increases in all of those conditions. Intervention studies have determined that lift tables, lifting hoists, lightening loads, and other engineering interventions can lower the risk of developing back injuries among workers.

The *revised lifting equation* results in two calculated values. The first is the *Recommended Weight Limit (RWL)* that corresponds to the AL in terms of acceptable weight of lift. The maximum possible RWL is 51 pounds. The second value is the *Lifting Index (LI)* that is defined as the actual weight lifted divided by the RWL. The LI gives a relative indication of the risk of injury associated with various lifting tasks. Available data does not allow prediction of the magnitude of risk for any individual or the exact percent of the work population who would be at an elevated risk for back injury as the LI increases above 1. The NIOSH perspective is that it is likely that tasks with a LI > 1 pose an increased risk of lifting related injury. Hence the goal should be to design all lifting jobs for LI of 1 or less.

As per Section 34 of the (Indian) Factories Act, 1948 (excessive weights):

1. No person shall be employed in any factory to lift, carry or move any load so heavy as to be likely to cause him an injury.
2. The State Government may make rules prescribing the maximum weights which may be lifted, carried or moved by adult men, adult women, adolescents and children employed in factories or in any class or description of factories or in carrying on in any specified process.

'Height Vertigo' or 'Height Phobia'

Vertigo can be described as abnormal perception of movement of the environment occurs as a result of a mismatch between the information about the person's position reaching the brain from the eyes. Vertigo is one category of dizziness (other categories are—faintness and miscellaneous head sensations). Vertigo is usually due to the disturbance in the vestibular system. Vertigo may represent either physiologic stimulation or pathologic dysfunction.

Physiological vertigo occurs in normal individuals when the brain is confronted with an intersensory mismatch among the three stabilizing sensory systems like car sickness, *height vertigo*, visual vertigo.

The most important diagnostic tool is a detailed history focused on the meaning of 'dizziness' to the patient. Is it faintness (presyncope)? Is there a sensation of spinning? Decrease in blood pressure, hyperventilation syndrome, hypoglycemia, somatic symptoms of a clinical depression, slight vestibular imbalance, etc. also can cause vertigo or other categories of dizziness. Appropriate investigations should be done to detect these disorders.

Emergency medical treatment of injuries and rehabilitation at construction site:

Trauma is the leading cause of death in most developed countries and is estimated to become the second or third most common cause of death across all age groups by 2020. Motor vehicle crashes are the most common etiology, accounting for the greatest number of injuries and deaths. Falls are the second most common cause of unintentional injury. It is clear that trauma is a large burden on the health care system.

Patients with blunt trauma frequently are encountered in the emergency department. The potential for early mortality and morbidity should be considered in all blunt trauma victims with a significant mechanism of injury. An organized assessment for life-threatening head, chest, abdominal, and pelvic injuries should be conducted with a recognition that definitive care may be provided after transfer to a certified trauma center. Proper stabilization measures including airway control, fluid resuscitation, and appropriate diagnostic studies should be performed prior to transfer. Airway control, assuring proper oxygenation and maintaining cerebral perfusion, are the hallmarks of early management of head injury. Attention to proper oxygenation and ventilation of patients with early tube thoracostomy is definitive in most patients with thoracic injury. Finally, pelvic stabilization and intravenous fluids are key management principles in abdominal and pelvic trauma.

Measures for Fracture

1. Do not move the injured unless the life is in danger from other cause.
2. Deal with the hemorrhage and breathing difficulties, if any.
3. Immobilize the fracture by the use of bandages using the injured body as support or by well-padded splint.
4. Immobilization should one point above and one point below. Remove the injured to the hospital.

Measures for Burn

1. Place the part under running cold water.
2. Cover the wound with several layer of sterilized cloth.
3. Artificial respiration if needed.
4. Immediate medical attention.

Measures for Wound

1. Stop the bleeding by anyone of the following methods.
   a. Direct pressure.
   b. Direct finger pressure into the wound in cases of larger bleeding wounds.
   c. Tourniquet (seldom needed)—use only as a last resort.

2. Avoid touching the wound with hands or unsterile material.
3. Clean the wound with running water and surrounding area with soap or spirit with clean gauze washing away from the wound. Apply ready-made adhesive gauze, bandage or sterile gauze and roller bandage as needed.
4. Keep the patient quiet; raising the extremity, if it is the bleeding part. Give no stimulants.

Cardiopulmonary Resuscitation for Unconscious Worker

Cardiopulmonary arrest is the abrupt cessation of spontaneous and effective cardiac output and ventilation. Cardiopulmonary resuscitation (CPR) is intended to provide artificial circulation and ventilation until other measures can be instituted so that spontaneous cardiopulmonary function is restored. Management of CPR is a team effort.

The scope of cardiopulmonary arrest and resuscitation has broadened enormously during the last two decades. Earlier it was confined to the management of unexpected catastrophes in hospital particularly in operation room. Subsequently it has embraced all the patients of 'sudden death' occurring both in and outside hospital with a systemic and uniform approach. CPR has now become a major public health endeavor involving a chain of personnel. The initial action starts by the lay persons around and is continued by paramedical personnel, nursing staffs, primary care physicians and finally by specialists and super specialists. Simple starting procedures 'mouth to mouth breathing' and 'cardiac massage', keep the patient alive and allow the further systemic approaches with equipment and drugs to act properly to give best resuscitation results.

CPR is further categorized as:

1. Basic life support (BLS).
2. Advanced cardiac life support (ACLS).
3. Post-resuscitation support (PRS).

Basic life support consists of:

1. Provision of a patent upper airway (A = airway).
2. Ventilation (B = breathing).
3. Well-maintained circulation of blood by closed chest cardiac compressions (C = circulation).

The ABCs of BLS can be instituted by any trained person without the need for specialized equipment. Regardless of the time from cardiopulmonary arrest to initiation of CPR, >6 minutes of closed chest cardiac compression is associated with increased neurological morbidity.

Provision of a Patent Airway

The aim of providing a patent's airways is to relive obstruction due to the tongue relaxing against the posterior pharynx. This is best relieved by head tilt-chin lift method.

Ventilation

Mouth to mouth breathing can provide adequate alveolar ventilation. Current recommendation: on initiating BLS, 2 breaths are given and then continued at a rate of 10 to 12 per minute. A single rescuer administering CPR should pause and give 2 breaths after each 15 chest compression (2 : 15). In two rescuers CPR, a single breath is to be given after every fifth chest compression (1 : 5). Exhalation can occur during the next compression.

Circulation

Circulation is provided by closed chest compressions and to be effective must be performed correctly. The most accepted theory (proposed) to explain how closed chest compressions cause blood flow through the circulatory system is 'cardiac pump mechanism' theory. This mechanism postulates that compression of the ventricles between the sternum and spine results in an increase intraventricular pressure, closure of the mitral and tricuspid valves and ejection of blood into the lungs and aorta. During the relaxation phase, negative intrathoracic pressure caused by expansion of the thoracic case, facilitates blood return and aortic pressure results in aortic valve closure and coronary perfusion.

Chapter

2

Industrial Hygiene

CONCEPT, DEFINITION AND IMPORTANCE OF HYGIENE IN INDUSTRY

Industrial hygiene has been defined as *"the science and art of recognizing, evaluating and controlling occupational health hazards"*. The word *'hygiene'* is derived from *Hygeia*, the goddess of health in Greek mythology. Hygiene is also defined as "the science and art of health and embraces all factors which contribute to healthful living".

Occupational hygiene is defined by the American Industrial Hygiene Association as *"that science and art devoted to the identification, evaluation and control of those environmental factors or stresses, arising in or from the place of work, which may cause illness, impaired health and well-being, or significant discomfort and inefficiency among workers or among citizens of the community"*. In simple terms, occupational hygiene is concerned with prevention of workplace diseases and ill health through anticipation, identification, evaluation and control of health hazards.

The role of industrial hygienist in the work setting is to provide expertise in identifying health hazards, using accepted instrumentation and methodologies to evaluate their magnitude and to provide advice on implementation of control measures. One aspect of that role is to provide information to the occupational health practitioners on the hazards posed by work processes. An effective industrial hygiene program must be proactive in recognizing potential hazards and setting up sound programs that reduce exposure hazards.

Planning and Conducting Industrial Hygiene Studies

While conducting an industrial hygiene study, the evaluation of the industrial environment is undertaken broadly: (i) To determine levels of exposure among workmen to various atmospheric contaminants. (ii) To determine the effectiveness of control measure. (iii) To investigate complaints, and (iv) For research purpose.

DIFFERENCE BETWEEN PERSONAL/DOMESTIC HYGIENE AND INDUSTRIAL HYGIENE

Personal Hygiene

The aim of personal hygiene is to promote standard of personal cleanliness within the setting of the condition where people live. Personal hygiene includes bathing, clothing, washing hands, toilet, care of feet, hands, nails, teeth, spitting, coughing, sneezing, housekeeping, smoking, eating, etc. Improvement of environmental health is a major concern of many industries.

Industrial hygiene is devoted to the anticipation, recognition, evaluation, and control of environmental factors or stresses arising in or from the workplace, which can cause sickness, impaired health and well-being, or significant discomfort among workers or among citizens of the community.

The objectives of health education in environmental health promotion through improvement of personal hygiene are:

1. To educate the people in the principle of environmental health with a view to bring about desired changes in health practice.
2. To secure adoption, wide use and maintenance of environmental health practice.
3. To promote active participation of the people to improve the personal and environmental health.

PHYSICAL HAZARDS

Heat Stress and its Control

The character of the thermal environment is determined not only by its total thermal energy content but also by the flow of thermal energy as a result of temperature differences. Operation involving high air temperatures, radiant heat sources, high humidity. Direct physical contact with hot objects or strenuous physical activities has a high potential for inducing heat stress in employees engaged in such operations. Operation involving high air temperatures, radiant heat sources, high humidity. Direct physical contact with hot objects or strenuous physical activities has a high potential for inducing heat stress in employees engaged in such operations. Such places include: iron and steel foundries, nonferrous foundries, brick-firing and ceramic plants, glass products facilities, rubber products factories, electrical utilities (particularly boiler rooms), bakeries, confectioneries, commercial kitchens, laundries, food canneries, chemical plants, mining sites, smelters and steam tunnels. Outdoor operations conducted in hot weather, such as construction, refining, asbestos removal and hazardous waste site activities, especially those that require workers to wear semipermeable or impermeable protective clothing, are also likely to cause heat stress among exposed workers. The ramification of human heat exposure is legion: they embrace social relationship, physical and mental well-being, and, ultimately, human productivity.

Five main medical disorders can result from excessive exposure to hot environments (in order of decreasing severity): heat stroke, heat exhaustion, heat cramps, heat syncope, and skin disorders.

A stable internal body temperature requires maintenance of a balance between heat production and loss, which the hypothalamus regulates by triggering changes in thirst, muscle tone, vascular tone, and sweat gland function. Production and evaporation of sweat are a major mechanism of heat removal (however, sweating causes loss of body water and sodium).

Heat stress is the amount of heat that is to be eliminated from human body to remain the body in thermal equilibrium and can be measured as metabolic heat load and heat loss or gain through the process of convection, conduction, radiation and evaporation. Heat strain is the physiological and pathological changes of the body due to heat stress. The equation of store (S) heat of the body due to heat stress is:

$$M + (R + C + K) - E = S$$

where M = metabolic heat, R = radiation, C = convection, K = conduction, E = evaporation and S = stored heat.

Effects of Heat Stress

1. *Heat stroke*: This is attributed to failure of the heat regulating mechanism. It is characterized by very high body temperature which may rise to 10°F and profound disturbances including delirium, convulsions and partial or complete loss of consciousness. The skin is dry and hot, classically, sweating is absent or diminished, but many victims of clear-cut heat stroke perspire profusely. The outcome is often fatal, even when patients are brought quickly to medical attention, death/case ratio of 40% or more have been reported. The treatment consisting of rapid cooling the body in ice water bath till the rectal temperature falls below 102°F. The rectal temperature should be monitored continuously, both to monitor the efficacy of hyperthermia treatment and to guard against the development of clinically significant hypothermia, which can occur if cooling is continued too long. Further, treatment is supportive and directed towards the many potential complications of hyperthermia. Hypovolemia, hyperkalemia, rhabdomyolysis, hypocalcemia and bleeding diathesis may require intensive supportive treatment. The patient should be kept in bed for several days until the temperature control becomes stable.
2. *Heat hyperpyrexia*: It is arbitrary to impaired functioning of the heat regulating mechanism but without characteristic features of heat stroke. It is arbitrarily defined as a temperature above 106°F. It may proceed to heat stroke.
3. *Heat exhaustion*: Unlike heat stroke, heat exhaustion is not because of failure of thermoregulation. It is a milder illness than heat stroke and is caused primarily by the imbalance or inadequate replacement of water and salt lost in perspiration (sweating) due to thermal stress. Heat exhaustion typically occurs after several days of high temperature. Body temperature may be normal or moderately elevated, but is uncommon to exceed 102°F. The symptoms, primarily dizziness, weakness and fatigue, are those of circulatory distress. It may be severe enough to require hospitalization, especially in elderly patients. Treatment is directed towards normalizing fluid and electrolyte balance.
4. *Heat cramps*: Heat cramps occur in persons who are doing heavy muscular work in high temperature and humidity when there is profuse sweeting. There are painful and spasmodic contractions of the skeletal muscles. The cause of heat cramps is due to loss of sodium and chloride in the blood.
5. *Heat syncope*: This is the common ill-effect of heat. In its milder form, the person standing in the sun becomes pale, his blood pressure falls and he collapses suddenly. There is practically no rise in body temperature. The condition results from polling blood in lower limb due to dilatation of blood vessels, with the result that the amount of blood returning to the heart is reduced, which in turn is responsible for lowering of blood pressure and lack of blood supply to the brain. This condition is quite common among soldiers when they are standing for parades in the sun. Treatment is quite simple. The patient should be made to lie in the shade with the head slightly down, recovery usually comes within 5–10 minutes.
6. *Skin disorders*: Prickly heat or miliaria is an acute, inflammatory disease of the skin.

The most practical and accurate criteria of physiological heat stress are body core (rectal) temperature and heart rate.

Heat Stress Indices

1. *Wet bulb globe temperature index:* ISO 7243 prescribes a standard method for the estimation of heat stress using three temperature measurements: those of a standard dry bulb, a wet

bulb and one inside a blackened globe of 150 mm diameter. The three temperatures are combined into the WBGT index using the following equation:

$$\text{Outdoor WBGT} = 0.7\,T_{\text{wet bulb}} + 0.2\,T_{\text{globe}} + 0.1\,T_{\text{dry bulb}}$$

Under this ISO standard, it is permissible to ignore the dry bulb temperature if there is little difference between it and that of the glob (e.g. indoors with title radiant heat load), in which case the equation becomes:

$$\text{Indoor WBGT} = 0.7\,T_{\text{wet bulb}} + 0.3\,T_{\text{globe}}$$

Portable heat stress meters or monitors are used to measure heat conditions. These instruments can calculate both the indoor and outdoor WBGT index according to established ACGIH Threshold Limit Value equations. With this information and information on the type of work being performed, heat stress meters can determine how long a person can safely work or remain in a particular hot environment.

Permissible heat exposure threshold limit value (ACGIH)

Work/Rest regimen	*Work Load (WBGT)*		
	Light	*Moderate*	*Heavy*
Continuous Work	30.0°C (86°F)	26.7°C (80°F)	25.0°C (77°F)
75% work, 25% rest, each hour	30.6°C (87°F)	28.0°C (82°F)	25.9°C (78°F)
50% work, 50% rest, each hour	31.4°C (89°F)	29.4°C (85°F)	27.9°C (82°F)
25% work, 75% rest, each hour	32.20°C (90°F)	31.1°C (88°F)	30.0°C (86°F)

2. *Corrected effective temperature (CET) index*: It is an arbitrary index which combines into a single value of the effect of temperature, humidity, movement of internal air and radiant heat on the sensation of warmth or cool felt by human body. Comfortable thermal conditions are those under which a person can maintain normal balance between production and loss of heat, at normal body temperature and without sweating.

Zone	*Corrected effective temperature (°F)*
Pleasant and cool	69
Comfortable and cool	69–76
Comfortable	77–80
Hot and uncomfortable	81–82
Extremely hot	83+
Intolerable hot	86+

3. *Heat stress index (HSI)*: It represents the percentage of heat storage capacity of an average man.

HSI	*Interpretation*
0	No thermal stress
10–30	Moderate to mild heat strain
40–60	Severe heat strain
70–90	Very severe heat strain
100	Upper limit of heat tolerance

4. *Predicted 4-hour sweat rate (P_4SR)*: It is a potentially very attractive approach to the assessment of heat stress is to attempt to relate it to the amount of evaporative heat loss required for thermal balance.

Zone	P_4SR
Comfort zone	1–3 L
Just tolerable	3–4.5 L
Intolerable	4.5+ L

5. *Psychrometric chart*: The psychrometric chart (ironically derived from the Greek *psychron* meaning cold) is a clear graphical way of understanding the effect of changing humidity and temperatures alone.
6. *Predicted mean vote (PMV) and predicted percentage of dissatisfied (PPD) indices*: More modern thermal stress may need to be assessed by these more complex methods than the simple WBGT index, as the transfer of heat by each physical mode is usually more sensitive to subtle changes. These indices are given in ISO 7730, based on measurement of air temperature, mean radiant temperature, humidity, air velocity, metabolic rate and clothing insulation.

Prevention and Control Measures of Heat Stress

- Adequate intake of fluid and salt
- Personal protection by means of body-cooling garments (microclimate cooling)
- Safe exposure time adjustment
- Administrative control of personnel, whereby the number and duration of exposures are modified by work-rest cycles or the provision of cool rest areas
- Proper ventilation and air conditioning
- Medical control through medical examination
- Physiological control through selection and acclimatization
- Clothing—light, loose and light color
- Rest between intense work
- Proper engineering design to achieve adequate cooling, ventilation, and shielding from radiant heat sources and/or to achieve a reduction in work rate through mechanization.

Engineering Controls

1. General ventilation: General ventilation is used to dilute hot air with cooler air (generally cooler air that is brought in from the outside).
2. Air treatment/air cooling: It differs from ventilation because it reduces the temperature of the air by removing heat (and sometime humidity) from the air.
3. Air conditioning: It is a method of air cooling, but it is expensive to install and operate.
4. Local air cooling: It can be effective in reducing air temperature in specific areas. Two methods have been used successfully in industrial settings. One type, cool rooms, can be used to enclose a specific workplace or to offer a recovery area near hot jobs. The second type is a portable blower with built-in air chiller. The main advantage of a blower, aside from portability, is minimal set-up time.
5. Another way to reduce heat stress is to increase the airflow or convection using fans in the work area (as long as the air temperature is less than the worker's skin temperature).

Changes in air speed can help workers stay cooler by increasing both the convection heat exchange (the exchange between the skin surface and the surrounding air) and the rate of evaporation.

6. Heat conduction: These methods include insulating the hot surface that generates the heat and changing the surface itself.
7. Simple engineering controls, such as shields, can be used to reduce radiant heat.

Personal Protective Equipment

A. *Reflective clothing*: It can vary from aprons and jackets to suits that completely enclose the worker from neck to feet can stop the skin from absorbing radiant heat.

B. *Auxiliary body cooling*:

   1. *Ice vest*: Commercially available ice vest, though heavy, may accommodate as many as 72 ice packets, which are usually filled with water. Carbon dioxide (dry ice) can also be used as a coolant.
   2. *Wetted clothing*: It is another simple and inexpensive personal cooling technique.
   3. *Water-cooled garments*: These are ranged from a hood, which cools only the head, to vests and 'long johns', which offer partial or complete body cooling.
   4. *Circulating air*: It is the most highly effective, as well as the most complicated, personal cooling system. By directing compressed air around the body from a supplied air system, both evaporative and convective cooling are improved.

C. *Respirator usage*: The weight of a self-contained breathing apparatus (SCBA) increases stress on a worker, and this stress contributes to overall heat stress. Chemical protective clothing such as totally encapsulating chemical protection suits will also add to the heat stress problem.

Administrative Controls and Work Practices

1. Training is the key to good work practice.
2. Hot jobs should be scheduled for the cooler part of the day, and routine maintenance and repair work in hot areas should be scheduled for the cooler seasons of the year.

Other Administrative Controls

The following administrative controls can be used to reduce heat stress:

1. Reduce the physical demands of work, e.g. excessive lifting or digging with heavy objects.
2. Provide recovery areas, e.g. air-conditioned enclosures and rooms.
3. Use shifts, e.g. early morning, cool part of the day, or night work.
4. Use intermittent rest periods with water breaks.
5. Use relief workers.
6. Use worker pacing.
7. Assign extra workers and limit worker occupancy or the number of workers present, especially in confined or enclosed spaces.
8. Pre-employment medical examination with physical fitness test.

Worker Monitoring Program

1. Every worker who works in extraordinary conditions that increase the risk of heat stress should be personally monitored. These conditions include wearing semipermeable or

impermeable clothing when the temperature exceeds 21°C (69.8°F), working with extreme metabolic loads (>500 kcal/hour), etc.

2. Personal monitoring can be done by checking the heart rate, recovery heart rate, oral temperature, or extent of body water loss.
3. To check the heart rate, count the radial pulse for 30 seconds at the beginning of the rest period. If the heart rate exceeds 110 beats per minutes, shorten the next work period by one-third and maintain the same rest period.
4. The recovery heart rate can be checked by comparing the pulse rate taken at 30 seconds (P_1) with the pulse rate taken at 2.5 minutes (P_3) after the rest break starts. The two pulse rates can be interpreted as follows:

Heart rate recovery criteria

Heart rate recovery pattern	P_3	*Difference between* P_1 *and* P_3
Satisfactory recovery	<90	–
High recovery (conditions may require further study)	90	10
No recovery (may indicate too much stress)	>90	<10

5. Oral temperature can be checked with a clinical thermometer after work but before the employee drinks water. If the oral temperature taken under the tongue exceeds 37.6°C, shorten the next work cycle by one-third.
6. Body water loss can be measured by weighing the worker on a scale at the beginning and end of each workday. The worker's weight loss should not exceed 1.5% of total body weight in a workday. If a weight loss exceeding this amount is observed, fluid intake should increase.

Medical evaluation of workers in hot jobs: Employees assigned to work in hot jobs should be medically screened:

1. Pre-employment medical examination: A good occupational medical history should be obtained.
2. Periodical medical examination.
3. Return-to-work examination after absence of >7 calendar days due to the illness and injury.
4. Special examination whenever considered medically necessary by plant management on an individual basis or on a physician's recommendation.

Ventilation

Ventilation is the process of replacement of polluted/vitiated air by fresh air. Industrial ventilation generally involves the use of supply and exhaust ventilation to control emissions, exposures, and chemical hazards in the workplace. Traditionally, nonindustrial ventilation systems commonly known as heating, ventilation and air conditioning (HVAC) systems were built to control temperature, humidity, and odors. Ventilation may be deficient in:

1. Confined spaces.
2. Facilities failing to provide adequate maintenance of ventilation equipment.
3. Facilities operated to maximize energy conservation.
4. Windowless areas.
5. Area with high occupant densities.

Problem Characterization of Poor Ventilation

1. Emission source:
    a. Where are all emission sources or potential emission sources located?
    b. Which emission sources actually contribute to exposure?
    c. What is the relative contribution of each source to exposure?
    d. Characterization of each contributor:
        i. Chemical composition
        ii. Temperature
        iii. Rate of emission
        iv. Direction of emission
        v. Initial emission velocity
        vi. Pattern of emission (continuous or intermittent)
        vii. Time intervals of emission
        viii. Mass of emitted material.
2. Air behavior:
    a. Air temperature.
    b. Air movement (direction, velocity).
    c. Mixing potential.
    d. Supply and return flow conditions, to include pressure differences between space and surrounding areas.
    e. Sources of tempered and un-tempered make-up air.
    f. Air change per hour.
    g. Influence of existing HVAC (heating, ventilation and air conditioning) systems.
    h. Effects of wind speed and direction.
    i. Effects of weather and season.
3. Employees behavior:
    a. Worker interaction with emission source.
    b. Worker exposure levels.
    c. Worker location.
    d. Worker education.
    e. Training and cooperation.

Objectives of Ventilation

1. To keep the air temperature of the workplace low enough for dissipation of body heat;
2. To prevent excessive humidity for evaporation of body heat.
3. To regulate the rate of air movement to facilitate loss of body heat.

Functions of Ventilation

1. To maintain oxygen content of the air and to prevent increase in carbon dioxide concentration.
2. To prevent any objectionable odor.
3. To prevent harmful concentration of dust, fume, gas, smoke, flammable vapor, moisture, and toxic pollutants.
4. To maintain reasonable conditions of comfort for workers.
5. To maintain body heat balance.

In short, ventilation has to perform three functions:

a. To supply sufficient quantity of fresh air
b. To distribute the air satisfactorily throughout the workplace
c. To maintain reasonable conditions of comfort for the operators.

The amount of ventilation depends on:

1. Size (including height) and type of room, building and its usage.
2. Duration and type of occupants and their activities.
3. Heat gains from the sun, hot processes, machinery and occupants.
4. Temperature conditions desired inside the place of work in relation to prevailing outside conditions.
5. The operation of the ventilation system.

Human Comfort Criterion

Optimum safe temperature	20°C
Optimum safe relative humidity	60–40%
Optimum safe airflow velocity	0.10–0.15 m/sec.
Floor space per worker	15 m^3
Floor area per worker	4.5 m^2
Fresh air per worker	20 m^3/hour
Air density	1.2 kg/m^3

Types of Ventilation

1. *Natural ventilation*: It occurs naturally through the openings of doors, windows, fanlights, skylights, and ventilators due to the effect of difference of temperature, specific weight of air, velocity, direction and pressure of indoor and outdoor air.
2. *Cross ventilation*: Cross ventilation can be obtained by the provision of large and suitably placed windows or combination of windows and wall ventilators for the inflow and outflow of air. Air movements of 45–60 m (150 to 200 ft.) per minute will be able to provide comfort to the workers.
3. *Roofed ventilation*: It is ventilation through ventilating areas in the roof by natural ventilation induced by due to chimney effect. The chimney effect is counteracted when the wind blows straight against these roof openings. Such interference can be prevented by suitably changing the design of ventilator openings. Ventilators can be of opening and closing type so that the ventilators on the windward side can be kept closed to prevent direct draughts of air interfering with upward flow of air.
4. *Mechanical ventilation*: Where ventilation openings cannot be provided due to surrounding buildings or due to the process carried on in them or large buildings where natural means fail, mechanical ventilation is resorted to. This can be done by either one or both of the following two methods:
   a. Ventilation through windows or other openings owing to the suction created by the exhaust air
   b. Positive ventilation by means of a fan or blower.
5. *Exhaust ventilation*: This can be effective by providing exhaust fans at suitable intervals in one side wall and adequate inlet openings in the opposite wall. Care should be taken to see that adequate inlet openings are provided so as to minimize draughts caused by high

inlet velocities and to avoid drop in the efficiency system. The total inlet area should be at least three times the total disc area of the fan. The exhaust fans should be provided with wind shields on the outside of the wall so that wind pressure may not decrease their efficiency. They should not, at the same time, restrict the free discharge of air. Windows and other openings near the fans should be kept closed as otherwise fans will draw air supply from these openings and thus cause short circuiting which is a very common fault with this type of ventilation. Exhaust ventilation can be provided in larger areas by having a fan of adequate capacity extracting air from the interior of the rooms by means of suitably placed ducting. Exhaust ventilation is often used in combination with natural ventilation so as to effectively ventilate work areas where natural means alone is not sufficient to provide adequate ventilation in all portions of work area.

6. *Plenum ventilation*: Plenum means 'overpressure'. In this system of ventilation, air is forced into the building by means of a centrifugal or other type of pressure fan and is distributed through suitably placed ducts. This system is useful where extraction system cannot be readily applied as in very large workplace or area. It has various advantages:
   a. Supply air can be conditioned.
   b. Prevents leakage of warm air from outside the building.
   c. Volume of air movement is many more times than that of exhaust ventilation.
   d. Better dilution of contamination.
   e. Lower worker exposure.
   f. Better circulation.

   Ducting should be such that the airflow should be direct at suitable velocities. Ducts should be smooth and straight as far as possible. Sharp bends and sudden enlargements and contractions should be avoided. Air velocities should not be excessive to the extent of interfering with manufacturing process or causing unpleasantness, but there should be a pleasant environment.
7. *Combined plenum and extraction system*: Better ventilation is obtained by this system by supplying appropriate quantities of air at suitable velocities at the required areas by plenum ducts and extracting the air into return ducts and sometimes recirculating this air after properly mixed with cool fresh air.
8. *Mechanical roof ventilation*: Mechanical roof ventilators are often used for augmenting natural ventilation in buildings where heat load is heavy. The openings within the area of influence should be closed to avoid short circuiting.
9. *Local exhaust ventilation*: In this system the heat from the source is removed by providing ventilated enclosures such as canopy or exhaust hoods by which heated air rises from a hot process environment. This minimizes temperature rise around the hot process. It has the advantage of preventing pollution of entire air space in a working enclosure.
10. *Emergency ventilation*: Where there is a risk of sudden outburst of explosive/flammable gases/vapors, especially in gas generating plants and compressor houses, this system is installed. This is usually of exhaust type ensuring at least 8 air changes per minute. During operation the temperature is lowered much below normal. Spark free axial fans are employed. Emergency ventilation switches will be on automatically when required.
11. *Air conditioning*: It serves to maintain a desired environment in respect of air temperature, humidity, purity and velocity regardless of the outside climatic conditions. It utilizes return air unless it presents health hazard. Self-contained air conditioners control temperature from 18–20°C and 30–70% humidity.

12. *Insulation*: The insulation of furnaces and other heat producing equipment will reduce the amount of heat exposure.
13. *Control of radiant heat*: In hot industries, the amount of radiant heat can be reduced either by lowering the surface temperature of the hot equipment (by insulation or by water cooling) or by radiation shielding.

Key Elements in Prevention and Control of Ventilation System

A well design system and a continuing preventing maintenance program are key elements in the prevention and control of ventilation system problems which includes:

Elements of a Good Maintenance Program

1. Establish a safe place to file drawing, specifications, fan curves, operating instruments, and other papers generated during design, construction, and testing.
2. Establish a program of periodic inspection:
   a. The type and frequencies of inspections depends on the operation of the system and other factors.
      i. Daily: Visual inspection of hoods, ductwork, access and clean-out doors, blast gate positions, hood static pressure, pressure drop across air cleaner, and verbal contact with users.
      ii. Weekly: Air cleaner capacity, fan housing, pulley belts.
      iii. Monthly: Air cleaner components.
   b. A quick way to check for settle material in a duct is to take a broomstick and tap the underside of all horizontal ducts. If the tapping produces a 'clean' sheet metal sound, the duct is clean. If the tapping produces heavy, thudding sound and no sheet metal vibration, liquids or settled dust may be in the duct.
3. Establish a preventive maintenance program: Certain elements of any ventilation system should be checked on a regular schedule and replaced if found to be defective.
4. Provide workers' training: Workers need to be trained in the purpose and functions of the ventilation system, e.g. they need to know how to work safely and how best to utilize the ventilation system. Exhaust hood do little good if the welder does not know that the hood must be positioned close to the work.
5. Keep written records: Maintain written documentation not only of original installation but also of all modifications as well as problems and their resolution.

Dealing with Microorganisms

If you suspect microbial agents, check for stagnant water in the ventilation system and prevent it as per the following measures:

1. Prevent build-up of moisture in occupied space (relative humidity of 60% or less).
2. Prevent moisture collection in HVAC components.
3. Remove stagnant water and slime from mechanical equipment.
4. Use steam for humidifying.
5. Avoid use of water sprays in HVAC systems.
6. Use filters with 50–70% collection efficiency rating.
7. Find and discard microbe-damaged furnishings and equipment.
8. Provide regular preventive maintenance.

Volatile Organic or Reactive Chemicals

If an organic or reactive chemical like formaldehyde is believed to be the primary agent in an IAQ problem, potential controls to consider include additional dilution ventilation, removal or isolation of the offending material, and the transfer of sensitized employees.

Tobacco Smoke Air

OSHA has published a proposed rule for IAQ (including tobacco smoke in the workplace), and this rule making is likely to be completed in the near future. Smoking policies should include provisions for dedicated smoking areas. Dedicated smoking areas should be configured so that migration of smoke into non-smoking areas will not occur. Such area should: (1) Have floor-to-ceiling walls of tight construction. (2) Be under negative pressure relative to adjacent areas. (3) Be exhausted outside the building and not recirculated.

Statutory Provisions for Ventilation and Temperature

The (Indian) Factories Act, 1948: Section 13: Ventilation and temperature:

1. Effective and suitable provision shall be made in every factory for securing and maintaining in every workroom:
   a. Adequate ventilation by the circulation of fresh air
   b. Such a temperature as will secure to workers therein reasonable conditions of comfort and prevent injury to health, and in particular:
      i. Walls and roofs shall be of such material and so designed that such temperature shall not be exceeded but keep as low as practicable.
      ii. Where the nature of the work carried on the factory involves, or is likely to involve, the production of excessively high temperature, such adequate measures as are practicable shall be taken to protect the workers therefrom by separating the process which produces such temperature from the workroom, by insulating the hot parts or by other effective means.
2. The State Government may prescribe a standard of adequate ventilation and reasonable temperature for any factory or class or description of factories or parts thereof and direct that proper measuring instruments as such places and in such position as may be prescribed; shall be provided and such records, as may be prescribed, shall be maintained.
3. If it appears to Chief Inspector that excessive high temperatures in any factory can be reduced by the adoption of suitable measures, he may, without prejudice to the rules made under sub-section (2), serve on the occupier, an order in writing specifying the measures which, in his opinion, should be adopted, and requiring them to be carried out before a specified date.

Industrial Noise

Noise is one of the most common occupational hazards in workplace. *Any unwanted sound is noise*. This is the most acceptable definition of noise defined by American National Standard Institute (ANSI). Noise may be classified as continuous (steady-state or fluctuant) or intermittent (impulse or impact). The characteristics of intermittent noise merge into those of continuous noise if the former is repeated very rapidly.

Several key terms describe the qualities of sound. The basic qualities of sound are:

1. *Wavelength*: The wavelength (λ) is the distance travelled by a sound wave during 1 second pressure cycle. The wavelength of a sound is usually measured in meters or feet.

Wavelength is important for designing engineering controls. For example, a sound-absorbing material will perform most effectively if its thickness is at least one-quarter the wavelength.

2. *Frequency:* Frequency, f, is a measure of the number of vibration (i.e. sound pressure cycles) that occur per second. It is measure in hertz (Hz), where 1 Hz is equal to 1 cycle per second. Sound frequency is perceived as pitch (i.e. how high or low a ton is). The frequency range sensed by the ear varies considerably among individuals. A young person with normal hearing can hear frequencies between approximately 20 Hz and 20000 Hz. As a person gets older, the highest frequency that he or she can detect tends to decrease. Human speech frequencies are in the range of 250–3000 Hz. This is significant because hearing loss in this range will interfere with conversational speech.
3. *Speed:* The speed, at which sound travels, c, is determined primarily by the density and the compressibility of the medium through which it is traveling. The speed of sound is typically measured in meters per second or feet per second. Speed increases as the density of the medium increases and its elasticity decreases, e.g.
   a. In air, the speed of sound is approximately 344 meters per second (1130 feet per second) at standard temperature and pressure.
   b. In liquids and solids, the speed of sound is much higher. The speed of sound is about 1500 m per second in water and 5000 m per second in steel. The frequency, wavelength and speed of a sound wave are related by the equation:

   $$c = f\lambda$$

   where c = speed of sound in meters or feet per second, f = frequency in Hz, and λ = wavelength in meters or feet.
4. *Sound pressure:* The vibrations associated with sound are detected as slight vibrations in pressure. The range of sound pressures perceived as sound is extremely large, beginning with a very weak pressure causing faint sound and increasing to noise so loud that it causes pain. The threshold of hearing is the quietest sound that can typically be heard by a young person with undamaged hearing. This varies somewhat among individuals but is typically in the micropascal range. This reference sound pressure is the standardized threshold of hearing and is defined as 20 micropascals (0.0002 microbars) at 1000 Hz. The threshold of pain, or the greatest sound pressure that can be perceived without pain, is approximately 10 million times greater than the threshold of hearing. It is therefore, more convenient to use a relative (e.g. logarithmic) scale of sound pressure rather than an absolute scale.
5. *Intensity:* Noise is measured in units of sound pressure called decibels (dB), named after Alexander Graham Bell. The decibel notation is implied any time a 'sound level' or 'sound pressure level' is mentioned. Decibels are measured on a logarithmic scale: a small change in the number of decibels indicates a huge change in the amount of noise and the potential damage to the person's hearing. The decibel scale is convenient because it compresses sound pressures important to human hearing into a manageable scale. By definition, 0 dB is set at the reference sound pressure (20 micro pascals at 1,000 Hz). At the upper end of human hearing, noise causes pain, which occurs at sound pressures of about 10 million times that of the threshold of hearing. On the decibel scale, the threshold of pain occurs at 140 dB. This range of 0–140 dB is not the entire range of sound, but is the range relevant to human hearing. Decibels are logarithmic values, so it is not proper to add them by normal algebraic addition. The decibel is a dimensionless unit; however, the concepts of distance

and three-dimensional space are important to understanding how noise spreads through the environment and how it can be controlled. Sound fields and sound power are terms used in describing these concepts.

6. *Sound fields:* Many noise-control problems require a practical knowledge of the relationships between:
   a. A sound field (a region in which sound is propagated).
   b. Two related concepts: Sound pressure (influenced by the energy, in terms of pressure, emitted from the sound source, the distance from the sound source, and the surrounding environment) and sound power (sound energy emitted from a sound source and not influenced by the surrounding environment).

Sound fields are categorized as a near field or far field, a distinction that is important to the reliability of the measurement. The near field is the space immediately around the noise source, sometimes defined as within the wavelength of the lowest frequency component (e.g. a little >4 feet for a 25 Hz tone, about 1 foot for a 1000 Hz tone, and <7 inches for a 2000 Hz tone). Sound pressure measurements obtained with standard instruments within the near field are not reliable because small changes in position can result in big differences in the readings. The far field is the space outside the near field, meaning that the far field begins at a point at least one wavelength distance from the noise source. Standard sound level meters are reliable in this field, but the measurements are influenced by whether the noise is simply originating from a source (free field) or being reflected back from surrounding surfaces (reverberant field).

A free field is a region in which there are no reflected sound waves. In a free field, sound radiates into space from a source uniformly in all directions. The sound pressure produced by the source is the same in every direction at equal distances from the point source. As a principle of physics, the sound pressure level decreases 6 dB each time the distance from the point source is doubled. This is a common way of expressing the inverse-square law in acoustics. Free field conditions are necessary for certain tests, where outdoor measurements are often impractical. Some tests need to be performed in special rooms called free field or anechoic (echo-free) chambers, which have sound-absorbing walls, floors and ceilings that reflect practically no sound.

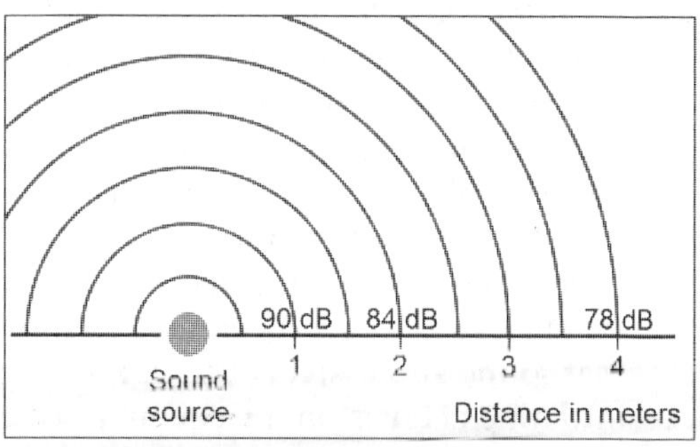

Fig. 2.1: Sound pressure level in a free field

In spaces defined by walls, however, sound fields are more complex. When sound-reflecting objects such as walls or machinery are introduced into the sound field, the wave picture changes completely. Sound reverberates, reflecting back into the room rather than continuing to spread away from the source. Most industrial operations and many construction tasks occur under these conditions. The net result is a change in the intensity of the sound. The sound pressure does not decrease as rapidly as it would in a free field. In other words, it decreases by <6 dB each time the distance from the sound source doubles. Far from the noise source, unless the boundaries are very absorbing, the reflected sound dominates. This region is called the reverberant field. If the sound pressure levels in a reverberant field are uniform throughout the room, and the sound waves travel in all directions with equal probability, the sound is said to be diffuse. In actual practice, however, perfectly free fields and reverberant fields rarely exist, most sound fields are something in between.

7. *Sound power:* Sound power is an equally concept like sound pressure. Sound power, usually measured in watts, is the amount of energy per unit of time that radiates from the source in the form of an acoustic wave. Generally, sound power cannot be measured directly, but modern instruments make it possible to measure the output at a point that is a known distance from the source.

   Understanding the relationship between sound pressure and sound power is essential to predicting what noise problems will be created when particular sound sources are placed in working environments. An important consideration might be how close workers will be working to the source of sound. As a general rule, doubling the sound power increases the noise level by 3 dB.

   A sound power radiates from the source in free space; it is distributed over a spherical surface so that at any given point, there exists a certain sound power per unit area. This is designated as intensity, I, and is expressed in units of watts per square meter. Sound intensity is heard as loudness, which can be perceived differently depending on the individual and his or her distance from the source and the characteristics of the surrounding space. As the distance from the sound source increases, the sound intensity decreases. The sound power coming from the source remains constant, but the spherical space over which the power is spread increases—so the power is less intense. In other words, the sound power level of the source is independent of the environment. However, the sound pressure level at some distance, r, from the source depends on that distance and the sound-absorbing characteristics of the environment.

8. *Filtering:* Most noise is not a pure tone, but rather consists of many frequencies simultaneously emitted from the source. To properly present the total noise of a source, it is usually necessary to break it down into its frequency components. One reason for this is that people react differently to low-frequency and high-frequency sounds. Additionally, for the same sound pressure level, high-frequency noise is much more disturbing and more capable of producing hearing loss that low-frequency noise. Engineering solutions to reduce or control noise are different for low-frequency and high-frequency noise. As a general guideline, low-frequency noise is more difficult to control. Certain instruments that measure sound level can determine the frequency distribution of a sound by passing that sound successively through several different electronic filters that separate the sound into nine octaves on a frequency scale. Two of the most common reasons for filtering a sound include (i) determining its most prevalent frequencies (or octaves) to help engineers better know how to control the sound, and (ii) adjusting the sound level reading using one of several available weighting methods. These weighting methods (e.g. the A-weighted network or scale) are intended to indicate perceived loudness and provide a rating of industrial noise that indicates the impact that particular noise has on human hearing.

9. *Combining and averaging sound levels:* Decibels are measures using a logarithmic scale, which means decibels cannot be added arithmetically. For example, if two noise sources are each producing 90 dB right next to each other, the combined noise sound level will be 93 dB, as opposed to 180 dB. The following equation should be used to calculate the sum of sound pressure levels, sound intensity levels or sound power levels.

$$\text{Total} = 10 \times \log_{10}\left(\sum_{1}^{n} 10^{\text{LN}/10}\right)$$

Often, using this equation to quickly sum sound levels when there is no calculator or computer available is difficult. The following table can be used to estimate a sum of various sound levels:

Difference between two levels	*Amount to add to higher level to find the sum*
0–2 dB	3 dB
3–4 dB	2 dB
5–9 dB	1 dB
10 dB +	0 dB

Example: There are three noise sources immediately adjacent to one another, each producing a sound level of 95 dB. The combined sound level can be found using the table above. The difference between the first two noise sources is 0 dB, which means the sum will be 95 + 3 = 98 dB. The difference between 98 dB and the remaining noise source (95 dB) is 3, which means the sum will be 98 + 2 = 100 dB.

10. *Octave bands (frequency bands):* Octave bands, a type of frequency band, are a convenient way to measure and describe the various frequencies that are part of a sound. A frequency band is said to be an octave in width when its upper band-edge frequency, f_2, is twice the lower band-edge frequency.
11. *Loudness and weighting networks:* Loudness is the subjective human response to sound. It depends primarily on sound pressure but is also influenced by frequency. Three internationally standardized characteristics are used for sound measurement: weighting networks A, C, and Z (or 'zero' weighting). The A and C weighting networks are the sound level meter's means of responding to some frequencies more than others. The very low frequencies are discriminated against (attenuated) quite severely by the A-network and hardly attenuated at all by the C-network. Sound levels (dB) measured using these weighting scales are designated by the appropriate letter (i.e. dBA or dBC). The A-weighted sound level measurement is thought to provide a rating of industrial noise that indicates the injurious effects such noise has on human hearing and has been adopted by OSHA in its noise standards. In contrast, the Z-weighted measurement is an unweighted scale (introduced as an international standard in 2003), which provides a flat response across the entire frequency spectrum from 20–20,000 Hz. The C-weighted scale is used as an alternative to the Z-weighted measurement (on older sound level meters on which Z-weighting is not an option), particularly for characterizing low-frequency sounds capable of inducing vibrations in buildings or other structures. A previous B-weighted scale is no longer used.

   A-weighted sound level: A person's ability to hear a sound depends greatly on the frequency composition of the sound. People hear sounds most readily when the predominant sound energy occurs at frequencies between 1000 and 6000 Hz. Sounds at frequencies above 10,000 Hz, such as high-pitched hissing, are much more difficult to hear, as are sounds at frequencies below about 100 Hz, a low rumble, e.g. to measure sound on a scale that approximates the way it is heard by most people, more emphasis must be given to the frequencies that people hear more easily. The most commonly used scales on sound level meters are the C scale, which give a flat, equally weighted response across the entire spectrum, and the A scale, which gives less emphasis to low-frequency sounds. The

A scale is often used in noise measurements, since it provides more weight to the annoying high frequencies. A sound level meter's A-weighting network is thought to rate most industrial broad-band noises much the same as the human ear does. Because of its simplicity and accuracy in rating hearing hazards, the A-weighted sound level has become the method recommended for measuring noise exposure by the American Conference of Governmental Industrial Hygienists (ACGIH) as well as the US Department of Labour as part of the Occupational Safety and Health Regulations.

Permissible Exposure Limit of Noise—OSHA Standard

Under Occupational Safety and Health Administration (OSHA) standard, workers are not permitted to be exposed to an 8-hours TWA equal to or >90 dBA. OSHA uses a 5-dBA exchange rate, meaning the noise level doubles with each additional 5 dBA. The following chart shows how long workers are permitted to be exposed to specific noise levels:

Permissible duration (hours per day)	*Sound level (dBA)*
16	85
8	90
4	95
2	100
1½	102
1	105
½	110
¼ or less	115

Schedule XXIV of Indian Factories Act, 1948, operation involving high noise (Model Factories Rules 120 under Section 87): According to this schedule.

Permissible exposure of continuous noise

Total time exposure (continuous short term exposure)	*Sound pressure level in or a number of dBA per day, in hours*
8	85
6	87
4	90
3	92
2	95
1½	97
1	100
$^3/_4$	102
½	105
¼	110

Note: 1. No exposure in excess of 110 dBA is to be permitted.
2. For any period of exposure falling in between any figure and the next higher or lower figure as indicated in column 1, the permissible sound pressure level is to be determined by extrapolation on a proportionate basis.

Permissible exposure levels of impulsive or impact noise	
Peak sound pressure level in dBA	*Permitted number of impulse or impact per day*
140	100
135	315
130	1000
125	3160
120	10000

Note: 1. No exposure in excess of 140 dBA is to be permitted.
2. For any peak sound pressure level falling in between any figure and the next higher or lower figure as indicated in column 1, the permitted number of impulses or impacts per day is to be determined by extrapolation on a proportionate basis

Instruments for Ambient Noise Measurement

There is a wide variety of instrumentation available for the evaluation of noise exposure, from very simple equipment to extremely sophisticated equipment used by acoustics engineers and consultants. Noise level measurements for steady-state or continuous noise should be made with a Sound Level Meter set to an A-weighted slow response or with an audio dosimeter of equivalent accuracy. For the measurement of impact noise (such as that from a drop hammer), an impact-noise meter with peak hold capability should be used. Sound level measuring instrument should be calibrated using an acoustic calibrator, preferably before and after the noise measurements. Instruments used for monitoring employee exposures must be carefully checked or calibrated to ensure that the measurements are accurate. Calibration procedures are unique to specific instruments. Employers have the duty to assure that the measuring instruments they are using are properly calibrated. They may find it useful to follow the manufacturer's instructions to determine when and how extensively to calibrate.

Health Hazards of Noise

Auditory Effects of Sound Stimulation and Hazardous Noise

1. *Noise induced temporary threshold shift (NITTS)*: The magnitude of a temporary threshold shift is proportional to the intensity and the duration of the stimulus and the recovery, unlike adaptation is slow. Recovery usually occurs within 16 hours, but take several days with higher intensities.
2. *Noise induced hearing loss (NIHL) or noise induced permanent threshold shift (NIPTS):* This is characterized by irreversible audiometric effects and pathological changes in the cochlea. The 4 kHz notch tends to deepen but also insidiously widens, encompassing adjacent high frequencies. Once the audiometric changes encroach upon the speech frequencies (2 and 3 kHz in particular), the effected individual becomes aware of the diminished acuity in his or her hearing. Speech discrimination with background noise becomes difficult and the associated tinnitus (which is highly variable in character) may become intrusive. The rate of progression again depends on the noise parameters cited previously and on individual susceptibility. Generally, progression at 4 kHz is initially rapid, but slows down after 10–12 years. Progression to involve the lower frequencies is associated with a flattening of the audiogram in the highest frequencies such that the characteristic notched audiogram is not a prerequisite for a diagnosis of occupational noise-induced hearing loss.

Characteristic of Noise Induced Hearing Loss

a. It is gradual
b. It is painless
c. It is bilateral
d. It may be either symmetrical or asymmetrical.
e. It is preceded by NITTS.
f. It is irreversible.
g. It is a sensorineural (perceptive) deafness.
h. In the early stage of the disease, speech range is not affected.
i. It depends on individual susceptibility.
j. Usually there is a notch at 4 kHz.
k. NIHL can be measured.
l. It expands in both the upper and lower frequency ranges when exposure is increased.
m. It is usually not amenable to treatment.
n. In audiometric test both air-conduction and bone-conduction responses are below the normal range and both are equal.

Non-auditory Effects of Sound Stimulation and Hazardous Noise

Sudden impact noise can produce startle reaction consisting of contraction of blood vessels, increased blood pressure, dilatation of pupil and both voluntary and in-voluntary muscles become tense (contraction). Vertigo, nausea, peptic ulcer, fatigue, increased pulse and respiratory rates, increased physical and psychological stress, irritability and socially undesirable behavior, reduced work efficiency and productivity, and increased accident and error—all are the effects of continuous exposure of noise in industry.

Noise and Solvent and Other Chemical Agents Interactions

Animal experiments have indicated that combined exposure to noise and solvents induces synergistic adverse effects on hearing. Experimental studies have explored specific substances, including toluene, styrene, ethylbenzene, and trichloroethylene. In addition to the synergistic effects with solvents, noise may also have additive, potentiating, or synergistic ototoxicity with asphyxiants (such as carbon monoxide) and metals (such as lead). Examples of relevant literature on interactions between noise and specific substances include:

1. Toluene (Brandt-Lassen et al., 2000; Johnson et al., 1988; Lataye and Campo, 1997; Lund and Kristiansen, 2008).
2. Styrene (Lataye et al., 2000; Lataye et al, 2005; Makitie at al., 2003).
3. Ethylbenzene (Cappaert et al., 2001).
4. Trichloroethylene (Muijser et al., 2000).

Audiometric Examination Procedure

Audiometry is the measurement of hearing. The results of such testing are recorded on an audiogram, a graph showing hearing (threshold) level as a function of frequency. Hearing (threshold) level is the number of decibels that the subject's threshold of hearing lies above the zero reference of that frequency. Thus, a pure tone audiogram compares the hearing of the person being tested with a standard hearing level considered to be 'normal' (i.e. the audiometric zero reference level).

A manual, pure tone audiometer is an instrument in which the tester has control of the frequency and sound pressure level of the pure tones presented to the subject. The employee whose hearing is being tested responds to the test tone by raising a finger or hand or pushing a signal button. The technician selects a particular frequency, presents short tone pulses with a tone-interrupter switch, manipulate the hearing-level dial to determine the subject's hearing level, and records that level.

Proper hearing tests imply use of adequate sound-treated hearing test room, carefully calibrated audiometric equipment, and trained technicians. Bone conduction pure-tone tests and air conduction pure-tone tests may all be required.

Hearing Loss Detection Formula

The formula for hearing loss compensation awards needs to be based on a reasonable cost of such a program to society. Damage risk criteria involve psychophysical, political, and socioeconomic considerations. Generally, these decisions are compromises between providing total protection, at exorbitant cost, and providing a reasonable amount of protection to a given segment of the population at costs that can be absorbed by the government, industry, and ultimately by the taxpaying consumer.

Hearing impairment can be described by three parameters:

1. The first parameter is the selection of the hearing test frequencies that will be used to determine the severity of hearing impairment.
2. The second parameter is the 'low fence', which can be defined as the minimum hearing threshold shift which has to be exceeded for legal hearing impairment to exist.
3. The third parameter is a scale for measuring the severity of hearing impairment based on a 'multiplier' of decibels of hearing threshold shift above the 'low fence'.

Procedure

The following procedure is used to convert hearing threshold levels into percentages of hearing impairment, according to the 1979 AAOO (American Academy of Ophthalmology and Otolaryngology) formula:

1. The average of the hearing threshold level at 500, 1000, 2000 and 3000 Hz is calculated for each ear.
2. The percent impairment for each ear is calculated by 1.5% the amount by which the aforementioned average hearing threshold level exceeds 25 dB (low fence). A maximum of 100% is reached at 92% dB (high fence).
3. The binaural impairment assessment should then be calculated by multiplying the smaller percentage (better ear) by 5, adding this figure to the larger percentage (poorer) and dividing the total by 6.

Sample of Hearing Loss Calculation

Following are examples of the calculation of hearing loss:

Mild to marked bilateral hearing loss				
Ear	*500 Hz*	*1000 Hz*	*2000 Hz*	*3000 Hz*
Right	15	25	45	55
Left	40	50	60	70

1. Calculation of average hearing threshold level:
   Right ear = (15 + 25 + 45 + 55)/4 = 35 dB = 15% loss
   Left ear = (40 + 50 + 60 + 70)/4 = 55 dB = 45% loss
2. Calculation of the hearing handicapped:
   Smaller number (better ear): 15 × 5 = 75%
   Larger number (poorer ear) = 45%
   Total = (75 + 45)/6 = 20%

Therefore, a person with hearing threshold levels shown in this diagram would have a 20% hearing handicapped.

Degree of ability to understand speech

Degree	*Average hearing level for 500, 1000, 2000 and 3000 Hz*	*Ability to understand speech*
None	Below 25 dB	No difficulty
Slight	26–40 dB	Difficulty with faint speech
Mild	41–55 dB	Frequent difficulty with faint speech
Moderate	56–70 dB	Frequent difficulty with loud speech
Severe	71–90 dB	Can hear only shouted speech
Profound	91 dB and above	Very limited usable hearing

Control Measures of Noise Hazards

Engineering Controls

The information collected during noise monitoring (particularly octave-band analysis, which indicates the sound level at selected frequencies) may be used to design engineering noise controls. Designers conceptualize possible engineering solutions in terms of the source (what is generating the noise), the path [the rout(s) the generated noise may travel], and the receivers (workers exposed to the noise). The noise control may involve the use of enclosures (to isolate sources or receivers), barriers (to reduce acoustic energy along the path), or distance (to increase the path and ultimately reduce the acoustic energy at the receiver) to reduce worker noise exposure. In general, engineering controls are preferred but are not always feasible because of their costs and limits in technology.

Administrative Controls

Administrative controls include:

1. Reducing the amount of time a given worker might be exposed to a noise source in order to prevent the TWA noise exposure from reaching 85 dBA.
2. Establishing purchasing guidelines to prevent introduction of equipment that would increase worker noise dose. While simple in principle, the implementation of administrative controls requires management's commitment and constant supervision, particularly in the absence engineering or personal-protection controls. In general, administrative controls are used as an adjunct to existing hearing conservation program noise control strategies rather than as the exclusive approach for controlling noise exposure.

Noise Monitoring

If there is reason to believe that worker noise exposure will equal or exceed a TWA of 85 dBA, then noise monitoring is required. A sampling strategy must be designed to identify all workers who need to be included in the hearing conservation program. The noise present must be characterized in terms of frequency (predominantly high, predominantly low or mixed), intensity (how loud it is), and type (continuous, intermittent, or impulse) using appropriate noise-monitoring instrument. Anytime there is any change in production, process, equipment, or controls, all noise monitoring tests must be repeated.

Noise Reduction

Noise reduction can be helped by the enclosure of noisy machines, the use of mufflers, damping, silencers, antivibration mountings, the treatment of reflective surfaces with absorbing materials, the limitation of the use of noisy equipment to times when it is required, and the distancing the workers from the areas of maximum noise.

Control of Noise Exposure (Provision of Personal Ear Protection)

Ear protection provides a system of attenuation of the incoming sound and thus minimizes the sound arriving at the tympanic membrane. Various types of protectors are available.

Plants having hearing conservation program generally assign their medical departments the task of fitting employees with ear plugs, ear muffs and hearing protective helmets. These personal protective equipment are frequently issued in the field along with general instruction on the need of good adjustment of the cushion to prevent leaks. Whenever personal protection is warranted, both the exposed employees and their supervisors should be convinced that ear protection is not only beneficial but also necessary to conserve hearing. The medical department has an important role in a hearing conservation program both in evaluation and protection.

1. *Ear muff*: Ear muffs fit over the ears and are sealed to the side of the head by a soft cushion seals filled with soft plastic foam or a viscous fluid. They are usually held in position by means of a headband but may alternatively be attached to a soft helmet. Attenuation may be 'frequency selective', protecting some frequencies more than others, particularly the higher frequencies rather than the speech frequencies. 'Amplitude selective' devices are designed to provide attenuation that increases with sound level. Such a device usually has a small hole which acts as a mechanical filter, allowing low sound pressures to pass but offering more resistance at high pressures. 'Active devices' incorporate electronic circuitry which limits the transmission of sound at high intensity and are of value when workers are exposed to short burst of high intensity sound or impulsive sounds. 'Anti-noise' devices incorporate circuitry which cancels out incident noise especially at low frequency. These devices are still largely experimental. Many of the newer muffs incorporate an inbuilt communication system.

   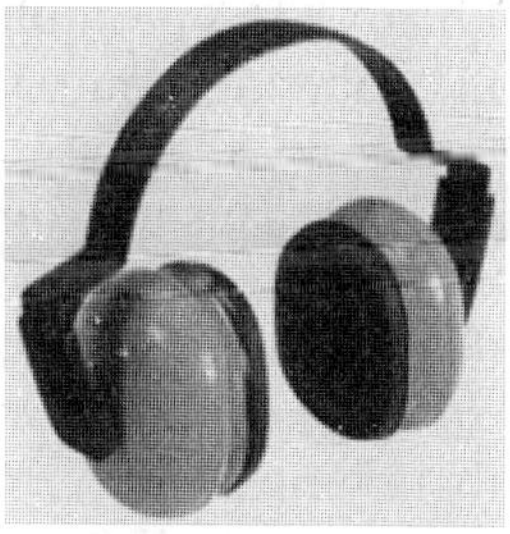

   Fig. 2.2: Ear muff

   While the ear muffs usually provide an effective level of attenuation, their value may be limited by any effect which decreases the efficiency of the seal, e.g. spectacle frames, goggles, beards and long hair, or scarves worm under the muffs. Furthermore, wear and tear may decrease the efficiency of the seal. It should also be emphasized that if protection is removed in noisy areas, even for a short period, the amount of protection will be severely limited. For example, if a protector with an 'assumed protection' of 20 dBA is removed for 30 minutes per day the actual reduction in noise dose received by the wearer will be only 12 dBA.

2. *Ear plug*: Ear plugs are generally thought to be less efficient attenuators of sound than muffs, but have the advantage that they are easy to use. They may be disposable or permanent. Disposable plugs are made of a compressible or conformable material. They are readily available commercially, but have a finite 'life expectancy' after which their effectiveness decreases. Permanent and custom moulded plugs have a longer survival, and are usually comfortable if made by an experienced technician. One of the main disadvantages of plugs is the increased propensity to otitis externa, although this too can occur with muffs. Dual protection with the use of both muffs and ear plugs may be indicated when the noise levels are extremely high (e.g. when L_{EPd} exceeds about 115dBA).

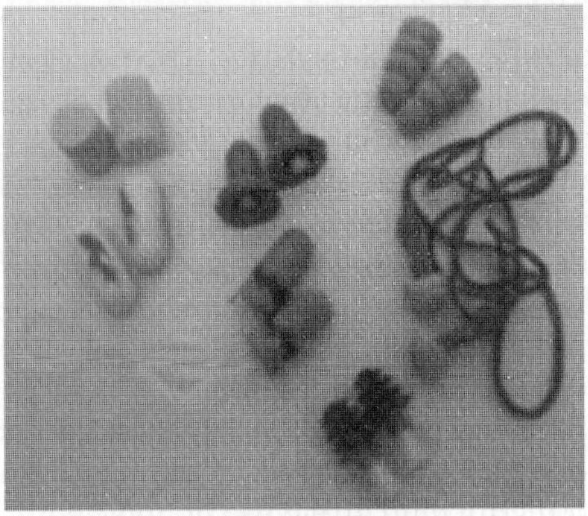

Fig. 2.3: Ear plug

3. *Hearing protective helmets (noise-excluding helmets)*: An extremely high levels of sound (e.g. in tunnelling), the protection offered by muffs and plugs, either alone or in combination, may be insufficient. Sound may still reach the ears through nose, mouth, eye sockets and the skull itself. The attenuation provided by the protector should comply with British Standard BS 510866 (ISO 4869), and the basic design features should comply with BS 6344. The 'assumed protection' of a device will vary with frequency and most will attenuate higher frequency sound better than low frequency sound. The 'assumed protection level' of noise exposure is obtained by subtracting the assumed protection of the device at each octave band frequency from the sound pressure level at each frequency.

Noise Reduction Ratings

When OSHA promulgated its Hearing Conservation Amendment in 1983, it incorporated the EPA labeling requirements for hearing protectors (40 CFR 211), which required manufacturers to identify the noise reduction capability of all hearing protectors on the hearing protector package. This measure is referred to as the noise reduction rating (NRR). It is a laboratory-derived numerical estimate of the attenuation achieved by the protector. It became evident that the amount of protection users was receiving in the workplace with the prescribed hearing protectors did not correlate with the attenuation indicated by the NRR. OSHA acknowledged that in most cases, this number overstated the protection afforded to workers and required the application for certain circumstances of a safety factor of 50# to the NRR, above and beyond the 7 dB subtraction called for when using A-weighted measurements. For example, consider a worker who is exposed to 98 dBA for 8 hours and whose hearing protectors have an NRR of 25 dB. We can estimate the worker's resultant exposure using the 50# safety factor. The worker's resultant exposure is 89 dBA in this case.

The 50# safety factor adjusts labeled NRR values for workplace conditions and is used when considering whether engineering controls are to be implemented.

$$\text{Estimated dBA exposure} = 98 \text{ dBA} - [(25 - 7) \times 50\#] = 89 \text{ dBA}$$

However, when assessing the adequacy of the hearing protection for hearing conservation (HC) purposes, we should only subtract 7 dB from the NRR.

Exposure for PPE/HC enforcement = 98 dBA – (25 – 7) = 80 dBA

Single/Double Hearing Protection

Dual hearing protection involves wearing two forms of hearing protection simultaneously (e.g. earplugs and ear muffs). The noise exposure for workers wearing dual protection may be estimated by the following method: Determine the hearing protector with the higher rated NRR (NRRh) and subtract 7 dB if using A-weighted sound level data. Add 5 dB to this field adjusted NRR to account for the use of the second hearing protector. Subtract the remainder from the TWA. It is important to note that using such double protection will add only 5 dB of attenuation.

Medical Evaluation of Hearing of Exposed Personnel (Audiometric Test)

When permanent threshold shift is recognized in a large number of employees from a certain noisy department, management must be informed of the problem and its consequences. One or more control programs should be presented. When the permanent threshold shifts are limited to a small percent of exposed personnel who show progressive and significant changes in hearing threshold, a decision must be made as to whether the employees should be removed from the noisy exposure. Such a decision is very difficult and must be based on complete evaluation of the individual, the environment and the economic implications to both the individual and management. In the final analysis, the decision to remove an employee from a given noise exposure is a management decision but the evaluation and recommendation of the plant medical officer will weigh heavily upon it.

Hearing Conservation Program

According to American National Standard Institute (ANSI), any unwanted sound is known as noise. Hearing, a precious sense which is responsible for effective speech communication can be damaged due to continuous exposure of high noise levels. In recent years, noise has become one of the major environmental pollutants mainly in industries.

Noise is not only a health problem but also a legal one as noise induced hearing loss (NIHL) in industrial workers due to industrial noise is compensable as per the Workman's Compensation Act. The compensation claims may amount to huge sums affecting the economy of the industries. Hence to safeguard workers from noise as well as to reduce compensation claims, "Hearing Conservation Program" plays a vital role.

The industries recognized the need for evaluating hearing and for preventing occupational hearing loss. For those industries having industrial medical program, the measurement of hearing threshold has been carried out by medical department personnel. The evaluation of the noise problems has involved not only medical and industrial hygiene personnel, but also management, safety, engineering, production, and maintenance personnel. The type and magnitude of the noise evaluation and control program may vary considerably, depending upon the nature of industry and the probability of hazardous noise exposure. The successful program must include the coordination and integration of four phases:

1. Physical evaluation of the noise exposure (noise measurement) and noise reduction.
2. Control of noise exposure (provision of personal ear protection).
3. Medical evaluation of hearing of exposed personnel (audiometric test).
4. Information and education.

Most manufacturing industries create some potentially harmful noise but the hazard will vary markedly with the type (continuous, impulse or interrupted), intensity and the duration of noise exposure. For that reason, each industry and plant must evaluate its own problem and organized its own hearing conservation program.

Physical Evaluation of the Noise Exposure (Noise Measurement)

The Relationship of Hearing Loss to Noise Exposure

With the development of accurate methods of measuring both the sound stimulus and the hearing level, more precise determination of relationship between hearing loss and noise exposure has become possible.

Control of Noise Exposure (Provision of Personal Ear Protection)

Ear protection provides a system of attenuation of the incoming sound and thus minimizes the sound arriving at the tympanic membrane. Hearing protective devices is considered the last option for controlling noise exposure. These are usually used during the time it takes to implement engineering or administrative controls, or when such controls are not feasible. Unless great care is taken in establishing a hearing conservation program, workers will often receive very little benefit from hearing protective devices. The best hearing protector, when fitted correctly, is one that is accepted by the worker and worn properly. If the worker exposure is above 85 dBA (8-hour TWA), hearing protection must be made available, along with the other requirements in the hearing conservation program.

Medical Evaluation of Hearing of Exposed Personnel (Audiometric Test)

There are two types of audiological criteria, to be applied to baseline and periodic audiograms respectively. A baseline audiogram is the first audiogram performed; in some cases, this will be a pre-employment audiogram. Periodic audiograms, performed yearly, are to be compared to the baseline. The criteria for referral for threshold shifts seen on periodic audiograms should be clearly distinguished from criteria for threshold shift used to trigger 'in-house' action by the hearing conservation program, such as refitting of hearing protectors or counseling.

Information and Education

Workers at risk of occupational noise-induced hearing loss need to be educated about the harmful effects of noise and the importance of hearing conservation measures. They need to understand the important of wearing properly fitting and appropriate ear protections. The attitude not to wear ear protectors must be changed. Workers should recognize and report the first symptoms of deafness, such as temporary threshold shift and tinnitus. Oral explanation, individual counseling, and lectures as well as leaflets, posters, films and videos may all be employed. Education must be extended to management so that their responsibilities are clearly defined, and managers exposed to potentially damaging sound levels must themselves be conscientious in their observation in safety measures.

Workers and management must understand the potentially harmful effects of noise to ensure the hearing conservation program is successful in preventing noise-induced hearing loss. A good worker's education program describes:

1. Program objectives
2. Existing noise hazards
3. How hearing loss occurs
4. Purpose of audiometric testing

5. What workers can do to protect themselves. In addition, roles and responsibility of employees and the workers should be stated clearly.

Training is required to be provided annually to all workers included in the hearing conservation program. Opportunities for maintaining awareness occur during periodic safety meetings, as well as during audiometric testing appointments when testing results are explained.

Typical case history of an individual with noise induced hearing loss: A 48-year-old man had chief complaints of constant, high-pitched tinnitus, and progressive hearing loss in both ears over the previous 2 years. He reported some difficulty hearing in quiet surroundings but noticed marked difficulty understanding speech in noisy environments. He did not report any previous serious illnesses, accidents, atypical drug use, or problems with his ears. For the past 8 years, he had worked in a noisy textile mill, where he said that he 'occasionally' wore hearing protective devices. The patient had not been exposed to other hazardous noises off the job, such as gunfire or motorbikes.

The diagnosis of NIHL comes under the domain of the audiologist.

Industrial Vibration

Occupational vibration reaches the worker through different paths or transmission routes. In 'whole-body vibration' it is conducted through a contacting or supporting structure that is itself vibrating like a ship's deck, the seat of a vehicle traversing rough terrain, a vibrating platform. There are vibrating work processes affecting the whole body in coal, iron ore and cement machinery that prevent blow holes in the final castings. In other industrial processes, the route of entry is through paths to the hands, wrists, and arms of the subjects, so-called 'segmental vibration' or 'hand-arm vibration'. The examples of hand-arm vibration are generated from pneumatic tools, electric-driven grinding, burrowing tools, rock drilling, and cross cutting timber. The prolonged use of vibrating tools and equipment can lead to a number of pathological effects. Physicians supervising a vibration-exposed work force should know the general principles involved in the recognition, evaluation, and control of vibration as a physical agent.

Occupational health professional needs to have some understanding of vibration measurement and its implications when assessing individual cases. Vibration is an oscillatory motion that can be represented by a simple harmonic sine wave with the properties of displacement, a velocity and acceleration. In practice, the wave is a complex, of differing frequencies and acceleration. Vibration can move in three orthogonal directions (x, y and z axes). They differ from when the subject vibrates from front to back (x axis) or from side to side (y axis) or in the vertical mode (z axis). To assess the medical effects, the accelerations and frequencies must be measured along the three coordinates of the biodynamic system proposed by the International Standard Organization (ISO), the British Standards Institution (BSI), the American National Standards Institution (ANSI) and the American Conference of Governmental Industrial Hygienists (ACGIH). It is the vector sum that is normally calculated (ISO 5349). The measurement of interest, in terms of biological effect, is the magnitude of vibration or 'A(8)' which incorporates intensity, duration and direction. The daily exposure to vibration of a person is ascertained using the formula:

$$A(8) = a_{hw}\sqrt{\frac{T}{T_0}},$$

where a_{hw} is the vibration magnitude in meters per second squared (m/s^2); T is the duration of exposure to the vibration magnitude a_{hw} and T_0 is the reference duration of eight hours (28800 seconds). A frequency weighting up to 16 Hz is factored into calculations to take account of the supposedly more damaging lower frequencies suggested by laboratory studies.

Segmental Vibration

Health hazards:

a. The hand-arm vibration syndrome (HAVS): The medical effects of using hand-held vibrating tools are more serious and more clearly defined than those caused by whole-body vibration. With the increasing technical developments since 1900, the use of vibrating tools has greatly expanded. Outbreaks of 'white finger' arising from both air-driven and electric-power tools were reported by Seyring, Hunt, Telford and Agate. Throughout the early literature this vibration hazard is described variously as traumatic vesospastic disease, dead fingers, spastic anemia, Raynaud's phenomenon of occupational origin, vibration induced white finger, and finally, since 1985, the hand-arm vibration syndrome.

b. Hand-arm vibration and muscles weakness: Patients suffering from HAVS are frequently noted to suffer from weakness of grip. The workers exposed to the use of vibrating tools frequently complain of weakness of grip and research studies have shown the vibration can cause damage to the small muscles of the hand and the nerves that supply them. The onset of weakness requires further investigation to identify any possible dose response. This will allow development of guidelines for working practice. All studies concerning grip strength need to be tightly controlled for age.

Workplace Health Surveillance

Workplace health surveillance is primarily for the detection of adverse health effects at an early stage. It can also be used as a means of identifying and protecting susceptible individuals at increased risk from the effects of hand-arm vibration. In addition, it can provide feedback on the effectiveness of control measures that have been introduced, and also, to prevent the progression of HAVS to the more severe and disabling stages.

Preventive and Control Measures

1. The vibration level or intensity and its spectral content: The known hazardous frequency range is assumed to lie in the 30–300 Hz. Recent research suggests that high frequencies partly neglected by a 'weighting curve' should not be discarded at the present cut off 1500 Hz frequency but are to be extended to 5000 Hz, when estimating HAVS dosage.
2. Vibration exposure time: There is a clear correlation between increasing impairment and deterioration with increasing vibration exposure time.
3. Continuous vibration, as opposed to interrupted work schedules, should be avoided; use 10-minute breaks or rest periods every continuous exposure hour.
4. An increasing grip force on tcol handles (coupling at the hand-tool interface) increases the vibration energy to the hand with greater damage to arteries, nerves, tendons, joints, and muscles.
5. The lighter the tool, the more energy is transferred to the hand since there is a less damping. Reduction in the weight in a hand-held vibratory tool reduces the workload on joints (elbow, shoulder) but increases the vibration.

6. Gloves are inefficient as protection from HAVS. Conventional glove designs provide little attenuation below 500 Hz. Gloves with built-in absorbent (damping) material is usually bulky, thus reducing manipulative efficiency. The absorbent material may in some designs actually increase vibration through material resonances.
7. As with all occupational hazards, there is an individual susceptibility. The so-called latent interval, the period between first exposure to vibration and the appearance of the first white finger(s) tip, is a valuable factor in assessing HAVS damage. The shorter this interval, the more hazardous the vibration. A subject with a very short latent interval compared to the mean of this vibration-exposed population is 'susceptible' to vibration effects.

Whole Body Vibration

Whole body vibration (WBV) occurs when the human body is supported on a surface that is vibrating. Vibration is an oscillatory motion characterized in terms of the frequency of the oscillatory cycle, its magnitude and its direction. The magnitude of vibration can be quantified by its displacement (m), its velocity (ms^{-1}) or its acceleration (ms^{-2}). However, it is usually expressed in terms of an average measure of the motion's acceleration [to give the root mean square (rms) value in ms^{-2}] so that a complex time-varying pattern is not unduly influenced by a few unrepresentative peaks. The rms magnitude can be related to the energy imparted and hence to the injury potential.

The frequency of vibration is expressed in cycles per second (Hz). The adverse health effects of WBV seem to be related mainly to exposures in the low frequency range, and frequencies below 3 Hz can cause motion sickness. Thus, to account for differences of response, current standard for exposure evaluation recommended weighting the frequencies of measured vibration according to the assumed deleterious effects of each frequency. Frequency weightings are applied to measurements taken in three orthogonal directions (x, y, and z-axes) at the interfaces between the body and the vibration.

Health Effects of WBV

The best-recognized health effect of WBV relates to the outcome of low-back pain (LBP). LBP is a symptom rather than a disease and consequently case definitions of outcome in research studies have varied in relation to anatomical distribution symptoms and in relation to their frequency, intensity and impact in terms of disability, medical consultation and sickness absence. Other health effects include radiating leg pain and sciatica and prolapsed intervertebral disk. Other suggested effects of WBV are neck shoulder pain or cervical disc degeneration, autonomic disturbance, disorder of balance and digestion, and effects on menstruation and perhaps labor.

There may be motion sickness include drowsiness, nausea, vomiting (often with little warning), stomach fullness, loss of appetite, facial flushing, dizziness, headache, inability to concentrate and sweating. It depends on the frequency (e.g. cycles per second) of vibration in Hz (usually below 3 Hz).

Factors Affecting Exposure and Control Measures

In addition to magnitude, duration and pattern of WBV, several other factors may relate to the injury potential, including individual susceptibility to injury, the dynamic response of the human body (mechanical impedance, vibration transmissibility, absorbed energy), body posture and health status. Dose may be related to the design of the vehicle, the cabin seating, the suspension, the road condition, the road speed and ultimately the behavior and training of the driver. It is required that the employer to assess and if necessary, measure the level of WBV to which workers are exposed.

Health Surveillance

Health surveillance, the result of which are taken into account in the application of preventive measures at a specific workplace, shall be intended to prevent and diagnose rapidly any disorder linked with exposure to mechanical vibration. Such surveillance shall be appropriate where:

a. The exposure of workers to vibration is such that a link can be established between that exposure and an identifiable illness or harmful effects on health.
b. It is probably that the illness or the effects occur in a worker's particular working conditions.
c. There are tested techniques for the detection of the illness or the harmful effects on health.

Preventive and Control Measures

a. Measures the vibration and evaluate vibration exposure time.
b. Adjust the subject's work schedule *vis-à-vis* vibration level.
c. Examine the ergonomic design (seat, instruments, control) with appropriate antivibration absorbent materials—advances have been made in 'air-ride' vibration isolators.
d. Institute pre-employment and periodical medical examinations with special reference to thoracic and lumbar vertebra. If the exposure is severe, X-ray examination is recommended every 4 years.
e. Undertake routine engineering maintenance.
f. Measure vibration of new plant machines, usually installed as replacements to increase production.

Improper Illumination

For any effective vision, the following light factors are essential:

1. Sufficiency: 15–20 foot candle is accepted as a basic minimum for satisfactory vision.
2. Absence of glare (excessive contrast).
3. Distribution: It should be uniform.
4. Absence of any sharp shadow.
5. Steadiness: It should be constant.
6. Color of light: There should be soothing effects on the eyes.
7. Surroundings: There should be a little color contrast.

Units of Light

1. Luminous intensity, which is the 'power' of a light source considered as a point radiating in all direction; this is measured as *candelas or candle power*.
2. Illumination or illuminance, which is the amount of light reaching a surface measured in *lux* per unit area.
3. Brightness or luminance which is the amount of light reflected from a surface measured in *lamberts. One foot candle is equal to 10.76 lux.*

Visual task	
Task	*Illumination in lux*
Casual reading	100
General office work	400
Watch making	2000–3000
Canteen	150
Engine assembly	300
Foundries	150–300

Color Coding

No light scheme can be fully effective without the proper color application. In industries, colors are used for:

1. Quality of workmanship
2. To reduce rejection
3. To reduce accident
4. To reduce absenteeism
5. To rise housekeeping
6. To improve moral of workers.

Adverse effects of color on health of people are mainly through its psychological effects.

Effects of color		
Action	*Color*	*Psychology*
Effect	Red and white	Stimulating
	Yellow	Freshening
	Orange	Tension producing
	Light green and blue	Relax feeling
	Purple	Depression
Size	Green and blue	Objects look larger
Space	Green and blue	Surface recedes
	Red and yellow	Comes forward
Temperature	Red and yellow	Warm feeling
	Blue and green	Cool feeling

Illumination

Illumination can be defined as the use of light to achieve the desired effect. These measurements are done during the day and at night depending on your work shift. Poorly illuminated work environments have health, safety and psychological effects on your employees and can result in injury, reduced production and increased stress levels.

General construction areas, ramps, runways, corridors, offices, shops, and storage areas shall be lighted to not less than the minimum illumination intensities listed in the following Table while any work is in progress:

Minimum illumination intensities in foot-candle	
Foot-candle	*Area of operation*
3	General construction areas, concrete placement, excavation and waste areas, access ways, active storage areas, loading platforms, refueling, and field maintenance areas.
5	General construction area lighting
5	Indoors: warehouses, corridors, hallways, and exit ways.
5	Tunnels, shafts, and general underground work areas: (Exception: minimum of 10 foot-candles is required at tunnel and shaft heading during drilling, mucking, and scaling. Bureau of Mines approved cap lights shall be acceptable for use in the tunnel heading)
10	General construction plant and shops (e.g. batch plants, screening plants, mechanical and electrical equipment rooms, carpenter shops, rigging lofts and active storerooms, mess halls, and indoor toilets and workrooms.)
30	First aid stations, infirmaries, and offices.

Poor lighting usually leaves the person with eye strain. It is also known as dimness of light. Eye strain is a very uncomfortable feeling. It can also get linked up with other eye related problem. If one spends more time working in poor lighting, the quality of his vision may start to deteriorate. Illumination is measured by Lux meter.

Health Hazards of Poor Illumination

Acute effects: Eye strain, headache, eye pain, watering from eye, eye congestion, eye fatigue, more accident, more error, less productivity, etc. Chronic effect is miner's nystagmus, a condition the mines workers suffered working with very dim light in the mines for a long period.

Thermal Radiation, X-rays, Ultraviolet Radiation, Ionizing and Non-ionizing Radiation

Ionizing Radiation

Ionizing radiation can be defined as a radiation which can penetrate the tissue and deposit its energy within it. Ionizing radiation may be higher energy electromagnetic radiation (X-rays and γ-rays) or energetic subatomic particles such as alpha (α) and beta (β)-particles and neutrons. According to their energy, X-rays and γ-rays interact with matter and tissue and although the mechanisms may be different, they all produce positively and/or negatively charged ions, which then interact with the absorbing matter to produce physiochemical changes by adding or subtracting electrons. The energy of these electromagnetic radiations will also determine their penetration, higher energy photons penetrating further than low energy one. When they do interact with tissues and cells, energy is deposited within the tissue.

The different radiations penetrate matter in different ways, the properties being determined by the size, charged and energy of each type; α-particles are stopped by a thin piece of paper or the dead layer of the skin, while β-particles can penetrate the hand but will be stopped by a thin sheet of aluminum; X-rays and γ-rays penetrate the body and an aluminum sheet, but are stopped by lead. Neutrons penetrate most materials, but may be stopped by thick polythene or concrete (hydrogenous materials); high energy neutrons have a high penetrance in tissue but low energy neutrons can be absorbed in the body because of the body's high water content. These overall properties of radiation affect the degree of cellular damage following exposure and the methods needed for protection.

Properties of ionizing radiation

Type	*Range in air*	*Range in tissue*	*Hazard*	*Source*
Alpha (α)	Few cm	10 s of μ	Internal	Plutonium
Beta (β)	Up to several mtrs	Few mm	External and internal	Caesium
Gamma (γ)	Many mtrs	Many cm	External and internal	Cobalt source
X-ray	Many mtrs	Many cm	External and internal	Hospitals
Neutron	Many mtrs	Many cm	External and internal	Reactors

Source: National Radiological Protection Board, Chilton, UK (now the radiation Protection Division of the Health Protection Agency)

Units of Radiation

The activity of a radioactive material is the number of nuclear disintegrations per unit of time. The unit of activity is a Becquerel (Bq). One Bq is equal to one disintegration per second. Formerly, the unit of activity was Curie (Ci) and one Bq corresponds approx. to 17 pico-curie.

The potency of radiation is measured in three ways:

a. *Roentgen*: It is the unit of exposure. It is the amount of radiation absorbed in air at a given point, i.e. number of ions produced in 1 ml of air. Now, Roentgen is being replaced by the new SI unit (International System Unit) to Coulomb per kilogram (C/kg). One Roentgen is equal to 2.58×10^{-4} Ckg^{-1}.
b. *Rad*: It is the unit of absorbed dose. It is the amount of radioactive energy absorbed per gram of tissue of any material. As per SI unit, rad has been replaced by gray (Gy). It is the unit of absorbed dose, defined as the dose of ionizing radiation that imparts 1 joule of energy to 1 kg of absorbed material. One rad is equal to 0.01 Gy.
c. *Rem*: It is the product of the absorbed dose and the modifying factors. It indicates the degree of potential danger of health. Sievert (S_V) is now replacing rem. It is the SI Unit of dose equivalent. The dose equivalent of 1 sievert is equal to 100 rems.

Health Effects of Ionizing Radiation

Somatic Effect (Systemic Effects)

a. Immediate effect: Ionizing burn, radiation sickness and acute radiation syndrome
b. Delayed effects: Leukemia (blood cancer), cancer to any part of the body (carcinogenesis), fetal developmental abnormalities and shortening of life.

Genetic Effect

a. Chromosomal mutation (sterility may develop).
b. Point mutation (gene is affected).

Permissible Exposure Doses

The radiation should not exceed 5 rad a year.

International Commission on radiological protection recommends:

a. 3 rems during any period of 13 consecutive weeks to the testes or ovaries, blood forming organs and lenses of eyes at any age over 18 years.
b. 235 rems of whole-body radiation for persons occupationally exposed from 18 to 65 years of age.

Hazards of X-ray and Gama Radiations

They are electromagnetic radiations of energy. They are used for material inspections in industries and welding checks. They have power of high penetration and are very dangerous. They cause burn, dermatitis, skin cancer, leukemia, fetal developmental abnormalities, and gene mutation.

Detection of Ionizing Radiation

Physical

Ionizing radiation cannot be directly detected by the human senses, but they can be detected and measured by a variety of means, such as photographic films, Geiger tubes and scintillation counters. There are also relatively new techniques using thermoluminescent materials and silicon diodes. Some of these techniques are used to measured individual doses on dosimeters (generally called film badges). Measurements made with such dosimeters can be interpreted to represent the energy deposited in the body or in a particular part of the body by the radiation concerned.

Biological

When a radionuclide is deposited in an internal organ, for instance via ingestion or inhalation, dose is generally calculated, because the activities are too small to be measured. The dose (or activity) can be assessed or measured by taking urine or blood samples and applying biokinetic models or be measured directly by special detection systems, e.g. whole body monitors. These systems are only available at special sites in the United Kingdom, such as British Nuclear Fuels, the Atomic Weapons Establishment, the Health Protection Agency, Sellafield Ltd or Harwell.

Principles of Radiation Protection

1. No practice involving exposure to radiation should be adopted unless it produces at least sufficient benefit to the exposed individuals or to society to offset the radiation detriment it causes (termed 'justification of a practice').
2. In relation to any particular source of radiation within a practice, all reasonable steps should be taken to adjust the protection so as to maximize the net benefit, economic and social factors being taken into account (termed 'optimization of protection').
3. Finally, a limit should be applied to the dose (other than from medical exposures) received by any individual as the result of all the practices to which he is exposed (termed 'application of individual dose limits').

Non-Ionizing Radiations

The electromagnetic radiation spectrum has been divided into a number of frequency regions. The most useful divisions are between ionizing (X-rays, gamma rays, cosmic rays) and non-ionizing radiation (ultraviolet radiation, visible rays, infrared radiation, radiofrequency waves). Non-ionizing radiation is that part of the electromagnetic spectrum which does not have sufficient energy to ionize matter, but can excite atoms by raising their outer electrons to higher orbitals, a process which may store energy, produce heat or cause chemical reaction (photochemistry). The non-ionizing radiation of wavelength below 300 nm is absorbed in cornea, 300–400 nm is absorbed in lens and >400 nm can reached to the retina. The wavelengths of non-ionizing radiation of major importance to the eye are grouped under the following headings:

Non-ionizing radiation	*Wavelength*
Ultraviolet	UV(C)—100–280 nm UV (B)—280–315 nm UV (A)—315–400 nm
Visible	400–760 nm
Infrared	IR (A)—760 nm–1.4 μm IR (B)—1.4–3 μm IR (C)—3 μm to 1 mm
Microwave	1 mm–1 m

The major and natural source of these wavelengths is sunlight which has a broad emission ranging from far UV (200–280 nm) to far infrared (3000–10000 nm). However, it should be noted that the eye is not normally exposed to the far UV component of the spectrum since this solar component is blocked by the atmosphere. In addition to sunlight, there is an ever-increasing amount of man-made candescent and incandescent sources which cover the full non-ionizing radiation spectrum.

Ultraviolet Radiation

Ultraviolet radiation exposure can occur from natural or man-made sources. Sunlight creates an important exposure for outdoor workers. Industrial process such as welding, plasma torch operations, and some hot-metal work produces UV radiation. UV radiation is also used for its germicidal properties in settings such as hospitals. Other applications include chemical synthesis and analysis, photoengraving, illumination, sterilization of foodstuffs, lasers, vitamin production, medical diagnosis and treatment and identification technologies. The UV radiation is subdivided into three regions: the UV-A from 315–400 nm, termed the blacklight region, UV-B, from 280–315 nm, the erythemal region, and UV-C, the region below 280 nm, the germicidal region. Wavelengths below 295 nm are absorbed in the epidermis, while longer wavelengths penetrate into the dermis. Wavelengths >300 nm are transmitted through the cornea and are absorbed by the lens.

Absorption of UV can produce photochemical reactions and result in effects including protein-DNA cross-linking. Some of the effects of UV exposure include photokeratitis and conjunctivitis, especially after exposure to wavelengths of 270–280 nm. Symptoms include pain, tearing, intolerance of light, visual haze, and a sensation of sand in the eyes. Cataracts have been produced by excessive exposure to UV in the 295–310 nm region.

Skin burn is also associated with exposure in the 300 nm band, with 297 nm wavelength considered to have the maximum biological effectiveness. Exposure produces the erythema or reddening of the skin we term sunburn. Tanning is also initiated by such exposure, with the migration of melanin pigment and resultant darkening of the skin. Long-term effects include premature skin aging with damage to connective tissue and the loss of elasticity that results in wrinkling (elastosis). More important is increased risk of skin cancers. The most serious of these, melanoma, often appears on body areas that may receive relatively less UV exposure such as the trunk or legs; it has, however, been associated with blistering sunburns received when young.

UV exposure can also create a photosensitization reaction if the individual has also been exposed to phototoxic agents, such as psoralens, coal tar, and some cosmetic preparations. Photoallergic responses mediated by the immune system can occur after exposure to pharmaceuticals, such as salicylanides, hexachlorophene, and certain antibiotics, as well as cosmetics.

Outdoor workers can use sunblocking creams as well as appropriate clothing (long-sleeved shirts, trousers, broad-brimmed hat, and/or neck shield) to prevent skin burn and tanning. Workers' eyes can be protected against low-sensitive sources of UV (low pressure mercury vapor lamps, sunlamps, and black light lamp) by use of glass or plastic spectacles, goggles, or shields. Lightweight clothing or UV absorbing creams will protect the skin. Exposure to low-intensity sources can also be controlled by limiting exposure time so that total irradiance on the eye or skin is controlled.

Sources of UV radiation such as welding arcs must be shielded from workers near the operation with use of materials opaque to UV to prevent 'arc eye' or 'flash eye'. For the welder who is directly exposed to the UV from the arc, use of personal protective devices including tinted goggles and face shields and densely woven or leather clothing will prevent excessive exposure. UV exposure for welders' helpers and other workers near welding operation can be mitigated by using shielding booths or curtains and by coating walls, ceilings, and other surfaces with pigment-based paints that have low reflectance in the UV range. Various types of glass and flexiglass shielding can protect against different UV wavelengths. Where these are not used, adjacent workers will require eye and skin protection.

The UV radiation produced by an arc welding can also initiate the chemical reaction that creates ozone and nitrogen oxides from oxygen and can decompose vapor of chlorinated solvents to produce highly toxic phosgene gas. The UV radiation control program must deal with these potential hazards as well.

Visible Radiation

Intense exposure from very bright short pulsed sources such as pulsed lasers and high intensity electronic flash lamps can induce thermal injury in the retina. Wavelengths in the blue range (400–500 nm) can also cause a photochemical injury in the retina. Shielding and exposure avoidance are the main controls.

Photic retinopathy may occur, due to photochemical damage by the blue light component of the arc welding, to individuals welding without eye protective goggles. In general, patients present with a decrease in vision which occurs immediately or soon after the injury.

Solar Retinopathy

Solar retinopathy is a well-recognized form of acute light damage caused by the direct or indirect viewing of the sun. Socrates advised that "a solar eclipse should be only observed by looking at its reflection in water". Galileo injured his eyes while viewing the sun through his telescope.

The quantity and quality of light available in the workplace must also be evaluated. Glare is a frequent problem where intensities are too great and where workers must view reflecting surfaces such as video display terminal (VDT) screens. Lighting must be sufficient for performance of the task but not so high as to produce glare or visual fatigue. Lighting criteria for different occupations have been developed for most work environments.

Infrared Radiation

Any hot body emits infrared radiation (IR). Industrial sources of significant infrared radiation include furnaces, hot metals, dehydration equipment and equipment for drying and baking of paints and surface coatings and spot heating. IR is produced by certain lasers and medical physiotherapy equipment. IR does not penetrate below the superficial layers of skin; its effect is to heat the skin and tissue beneath it. Radiation in the near infrared region (0.75–1.5 μm) can cause acute skin burn and may result in increased skin pigmentation. Excessive exposure of the eyes to IR from furnaces and other hot bodies has traditionally been thought to produce "glass blower's cataract" or 'heat cataract'. Overexposure to near infrared may also damage the retina by protein denaturation. Chronic exposure to excessive IR can also cause a 'dry eye' irritation of cornea.

Reflective aluminum shielding and aluminized clothing are often used to reduce infrared exposure and thermal loading for workers at furnaces and other hot metal working operation. Protective eyewear and face-shields should be components of the protective outfit. National Institute of Occupational Safety and Health (NIOSH) noted that glassworkers, arc welders and other may be exposed to both UV and IR, necessitating use of special glasses that absorb in both regions of the spectrum. This specific hazard was studied by Okuno who developed a theoretical model of the human eye and its exposure to infrared radiation. Temperature distributions within it were calculated, suggesting that IR cataracts in the workplace result from the generation of heat by absorption of IR in the cornea and heat conduction to the lens.

Safe Infrared Exposure Levels

The available data indicate that acute ocular damage from the incandescent hot bodies found in industry can occur with energy densities between 4 and 8 Wsec/cm^2 (1–2 cal/cm^2) incident on the cornea. The ocular tissue involved would depend on the wavelengths that are absorbed. As these relate to threshold phenomena, it would appear that a maximum permissible dose of 0.1–0.8 Wsec/cm^2 (0.1–0.2 cal/cm^2) could limit the occurrence of these acute effects. A further reduction by a factor of 10 should prevent the more chronic effects of intraocular tissues.

Infrared and UV radiation filtration is readily achieved in glass filter with additives such as iron-oxide, but the visible attenuation determines the shade number, which is a logarithmic expression of attenuation. Normally a shade 3–4 is used for gas welding (goggles), 10–14 for arc welding and plasma arc operations (helmet protection required). The rule of thumb is that if the welder finds the arc to view, adequate attenuation is provided against ocular hazards. Supervisors, welders' helpers and other people in the work area may require filters with a relatively low shade number (e.g. 3–4) to protect against welder's photokeratitis (arc-eye). In recent years, a new type of welding filter, the auto darkening filter has appeared on the scene. Regardless of the type of filter, it should meet American National Standard Institute (ANSI) Z87.1 and Z49.1 standards for fixed welding filters specified for the dark shade.

Microwave Radiation

Microwave radiation is found in radar and communications equipment, diathermy applications, and industrial and consumer ovens. Microwave intensities can be sufficient to cause significant local heating of tissues. The effect is related to wavelength, power intensity, and time of exposure as well as body size, its electrical properties, and whether reflecting surfaces are present. Generally, the longer wavelengths will produce a greater temperature rise in deeper tissues than will the shorter wavelengths. However, the given power-intensity, there is less subjective awareness to the heat from longer wavelengths than from shorter wavelengths because of their absorption beneath the body's surface. An intolerable rise in body temperature, as well as localized damage, can result from an exposure of sufficient intensity and time. The eye, which has a limited blood supply to dissipate localized heat, can suffer lens opacities, cataracts, corneal damage and retinal lesions. Testicular lesions and decreased sperm counts have also been reported. Acute, accidental exposure of the eyes to microwave radiation may lead to skin burns, conjunctival infection and loss of corneal epithelium.

Radiofrequency Radiation

Radiofrequency fields (RF) are a segment of the non-ionizing part of the electromagnetic spectrum. RF range from a few kHz to several hundreds of GHz. The public may be exposed to RF produced by AM, FM radio and television broadcast antennae, navigations systems, cordless telephones, wireless local area networks and increasingly by mobile phone base stations and mobile phone handsets. Occupational exposures to RF may be experienced while operating and maintaining radio and television broadcasting and telecommunication systems. Additional significant sources of occupational RF exposures are dielectric heaters used for heating, sealing and melting vinyl and other materials and from military and civilian use of radar systems. In the medical field, exposures can occur from the use of magnetic resonance imaging (MRI), diathermy or electrosurgery. Workers in the electric utility industry may also be exposed to RF from antennae located on or near electric utility facilities. RF exposure in the far fields (at least several wavelengths away from the antennae) is typically measured as power density in W/m^2 or mW/cm^2. In near fields (close to the source of exposure relative to wavelength), exposure to RF is measured as electric and magnetic fields, in V/m and A/m, respectively. Since the actual amount of exposure, a person receives from an RF field is also dependent on many factors, such as body size, grounding state of the person and frequency, uniformity and polarization of the field, in addition to field intensity, the internal exposure is typically expressed as specific absorption rate (SAR) in W/kg.

Effects of RF

Exposure to RF radiation induces heating in body tissues and imposes a heat load on the whole body, thus thermal mechanisms are accepted and prevention of excessive heating (above 1°C) serve as a basis for most international guidelines. High RF may interfere with pacemakers and other implanted medical devices. Direct contact with or very close proximity to an RF source, through an electric arc, may result in severe burns which tend to heal poorly. The lens of the human eye, due to lack of circulation and insufficient mechanisms to eliminate thermal energy, is known to be sensitive to heat. Therefore, heating due to high RF exposure could result in cataract. Long-term exposure may produce some adverse effects include nervous, neuroendocrine, reproductive, immune and sensory system effects, including cataracts, decrease birth-weight, behavioral changes and change in blood cell concentrations.

Occupational exposure to RF radiation may exceed exceptionable limits for maintenance crews on broadcast towers and radar devices, operators of dielectric heaters, shortwave diathermy devices and microwave oven. Exposure should be reduced by engineering controls, such as total or partial enclosure to limit leakage, interlocks, and additional shielding where necessary. Other controls including limiting access to RF field areas and reducing power during maintenance operations. Present guidance on occupational exposure is based on restricting the RF-induced whole-body SAR to <0.4 W/kg (a safety factor of 10); a heat load sufficiently small that its contribution to other possible heat loads, generated from hard physical work and/or imposed by high ambient temperatures, can be neglected.

EFFECT OF HAZARDOUS EXPOSURE

According to the classification of hazardous chemical substances (HCS):

1. *Carcinogen*: A chemical is considered to be carcinogen if; (a) it has been evaluated by the International Agency for Research on Cancer (IARC), and found to be a carcinogen or potential carcinogen; or (b) it is listed as a carcinogen or potential carcinogen in the annual report on carcinogens published by the National Toxicology Program (NTP) (latest edition); or (c) it is regulated by OSHA as carcinogen.
2. *Corrosive*: A chemical that causes visible destruction of, or irreversible alterations in, living tissue by chemical action at the site of contact.
3. *Toxic agents*: Dose-response relationship is a useful indicator of the toxicity of a chemical. Toxic doses in man may range from µg to g/kg body weight and chemical may be classified according to their probable lethal human dose (LD_{50}):
   a. Practically non-toxic
   b. Slightly toxic
   c. Moderately toxic
   d. Very toxic
   e. Extremely toxic
   f. Supertoxic.
4. *Irritant*: A chemical which is not corrosive, but which causes a reversible inflammatory effect on living tissue by chemical action at the site of contact, e.g. chlorine, ammonia.
5. *Target organ effects*: The following is a target organ categorization of effects which may occur, including examples of signs and symptoms and chemicals which have been found to cause such effects. These examples are presented to illustrate the range and diversity of effects and hazards found in the workplace:
   a. Hepatotoxins: Chemicals which produce liver damage, e.g. carbon tetrachloride, and nitrosamines.
   b. Nephrotoxins: Chemicals which produce kidney damage, e.g. halogenated hydrocarbons and uranium.
   c. Neurotoxins: Chemical which produce their primary toxic effects on the nervous system, e.g. mercury and carbon disulfide.
   d. Agents which acts on hematopoietic system, e.g. benzene.
   e. Reproductive toxins: Chemicals which effect the reproductive capabilities including chromosomal damage (mutations) and effect on fetuses (teratogenesis), e.g. lead.
   f. Cutaneous hazards: Chemicals which can affect the dermal layer of the body, e.g. ketones and chlorinated compounds.
   g. Eye hazards: Chemicals which affect the eye or visual capacity, e.g. organic solvent, acids and alkalis.
   h. Agents which damage the lung: Chemical which irritates or damage the pulmonary tissue, e.g. ozone and chlorine.

Genetic Toxicology

Genetic toxicology is the study of how chemical or physical agents affect the intricate process of heredity. Genotoxic chemicals are defined as compounds that are capable of modifying the hereditary material of living cells.

Genotoxicity, Mutagenicity and Carcinogenicity

Genotoxicity of chemical agent is an intrinsic chemical character, based on the agent's electrophilic potential to bind with such nucliophilic sites in the cellular macromolecules as deoxyribonucleic acid, DNA, the carrier of hereditary information. Genotoxicity is thus toxicity manifested in the genetic material of cells. The definition of genotoxicity as discussed in a report of IARC (1992) is broad and include both direct and indirect effects in DNA:

1. The induction of mutation (gene, chromosomal, genomial, recombinational) that at the molecular level are similar to events known to be involved in carcinogenesis.
2. Indirect surrogate events associated with mutagenesis (e.g. unscheduled DNA synthesis and sister chromatid exchange).
3. DNA damage (e.g. the formation of adducts), which may eventually lead to mutation.

Mutations are permanent hereditary changes in the cell lines, either horizontally in the somatic cells or vertically in the germinal (sex) cells of the body. That is, mutations may affect the organism itself through changes in body cells, or they may be passed onto other generations through alteration of the sex cells. Genotoxicity thus precedes mutagenicity although most of genotoxicity is repaired and is never expressed as mutations. Somatic mutations are induced at the cellular level and in the event that they lead to cell death or malignancies, may become manifest as various disorders of tissues or of the organism itself. Somatic mutations are thought to be related to aging effects or to the induction of atherosclerotic plaque, mutation in the germ cell line may be transferred to the zygote, the fertilized egg cell, and be expressed in the offspring generation. The most important mutational disorders found in the newborn are induced by mal-segregation of chromosomes during gametogenesis and result in severe chromosomal syndromes (e.g. trisomy 21 or Down's syndrome and monosomy X or Turner's syndrome). The relationship of genotoxicity to carcinogenicity is well supported.

Immunotoxicology

Immunotoxicology has been defined as the discipline concerned with the study of the events that can lead to undesired effects as a result of interaction of xenobiotics with the immune system. These undesired events may result as a consequence of (1) a direct and/or indirect effect of the xenobiotic on the immune system, or (2) as immunologically based host response to the compound and/or its metabolites or host antigens modified by the compound or its metabolites.

PREVENTION AND CONTROL OF AIR POLLUTION

Cyclones

Cyclones operate to collect relatively large size particulate matter from a gaseous stream using centrifugal forces. Dust laden gas is made to rotate in a decreasing diameter pathway forcing solids to the outer edge of the gas stream for deposition into the bottom of the cyclone. Efficiencies of 90% in particle sizes of 10 μ or greater are possible.

Incinerators

Incineration involves the high efficiency combustion of certain solid, liquid, or gaseous wastes. The reactions may be self-sustaining based on the combustibility of the waste or require the addition of fuels. They may be batch operations or continuous as with flares used to burn off methane from landfills; and, they may incorporate secondary control methods and operate at efficiency levels of 99.99%, as with hazardous waste incinerators. Combustion temperatures, contact time, and mass transfer are the major parameters affecting incineration performance.

Absorption and Wet Scrubbing Equipment

The goal in absorption and wet scrubbing equipment is the removal of gases and particulate matter from an exhaust stream by causing the gaseous contamination to become dissolved into the liquid stream and the solids to be entrained in the liquid. The rate of gas transfer into the liquid is dependent upon the solubility, mass transfer mechanism, and equilibrium concentration of the gas in solution. Gas collection efficiencies in the range of 99% are possible. The rate of particulate matter collection at constant pressure drops is inversely proportional to the aerodynamic mean diameter of the particulate matter and scrubber droplets.

Baghouses

Baghouses utilize sieving, impaction, agglomeration, and electrostatic filtration principles to remove solids from a gaseous exhaust stream. Baghouses maximize the filtration area by configuring the fabric filter media into a series of long small-diameter fabric tubes referred to as bags. They are tightly packed into a housing wherein the dust laden air moves across the bag fabric thereby removing it from the gas stream and building up a filter cake which further enhances air cleaning. The filter cake is removed to hoppers by various shaking means.

Electrostatic Precipitators

This control device utilizes gaseous ions to charge particles which are then moved through an electric field to be deposited onto charged collection plates. Collected particulate material is then removed by rapping or washing of the plates. To produce the free ions and electric field, high internal voltages are required. Since the collection process does not rely on mechanical processes such as sieving or impaction, but rather electrostatic forces, the internal gas passages within a precipitator are relatively open with small pressure drops and lower energy costs to move the gas stream. High collection efficiencies are possible, but collecting efficiency may drastically change with changes in operating parameters.

Adsorption

The process of adsorption involves the molecular attraction of gas phase materials onto the surface of certain solids. This attraction may be chemical or physical in nature and is predominantly a surface effect. Certain materials like activated carbon charcoal possess the large internal surface area and the presence of physical attraction forces to adsorb large quantities of certain gases within their structure. The rate of adsorption is affected by the temperature, concentration, atmospheric pressure, and molecular structure of the gas.

Cyclone Separator

Cyclonic separation is a method of removing *particulates* from an air (or gas) stream, without the use of *filters*, through *vortex* separation. Rotational effects and gravity are used to separate mixtures of solids and fluids. A high-speed rotating airflow is established within a cylindrical or conical container called a cyclone. Airflows in a spiral pattern, beginning at the top (wide end) of the cyclone and ending at the bottom (narrow) end before exiting the cyclone in a straight stream through the center of the cyclone and out the top. Larger (denser) particles in the rotating airstream have too much inertia to follow the tight curve of the airstream and strike the outside wall, falling then to the bottom of the cyclone where they can be removed. In a conical system, as the rotating airflow moves towards the narrow end of the cyclone the rotational radius of the airstream is reduced, separating smaller and smaller particles from the airstream. The cyclone geometry, together with airflow rate, defines the *cut point* of the cyclone. This is the size of particle that will be removed from the airstream with a 50% efficiency. Particles larger than the cut point will be removed with a greater efficiency, and smaller particles with a lower efficiency. Large scale cyclones are used in *sawmills* to remove sawdust from extracted air. Cyclones are also used in *oil-refineries* to separate oils and gases, and in the *cement* industry as components of *kiln* preheaters.

Fabric Filters

Commonly known as baghouses, fabric collectors use filtration to separate dust particulates from dusty gases. They are one of the most efficient and cost-effective types of dust collectors available and can achieve a collection efficiency of >99% for very fine particulates. Dust-laden gases enter the baghouse and pass through fabric bags that act as filters. The bags can be of woven or felted cotton, synthetic, or glass fiber material in either a tube or envelope shape. The high efficiency of these collectors is due to the dust cake formed on the surfaces of the bags. The fabric primarily provides a surface on which dust particulates collect through the following four mechanisms:

a. Inertial collection: Dust particles strike the fibers placed perpendicular to the gas flow direction instead of changing direction with the gas stream.
b. Interception: Particles that do not cross the fluid streamlines come in contact with fibers because of the fiber size.
c. Brownian movement: Sub-micrometre particles are diffused, increasing the probability of contact between the particles and collecting surfaces.
d. Electrostatic forces: The presence of an electrostatic charge on the particles and the filter can increase dust capture. A combination of these mechanisms results in formation of the dust cake on the filter, which eventually increases the resistance to gas flow. The filter must be cleaned periodically.

SAMPLING OF AIRBORNE CONTAMINANTS

To have representative samples the following basic question must be answered:

1. Where to sample—location.
2. How long to sample—duration.
3. How many samples—number.
4. When to sample—covering typical operations

The above four questions are discussed below:

1. Samples are usually collected in the following areas:
   a. At the breathing zone of the worker.
   b. In the general atmosphere of the room.
   c. At an operation itself.

If the purpose is to calculate the average weighted daily exposure the samples are collected in the breathing zone and in the general room air when the purpose is to define potential hazard. Check compliance with regulations or obtain data for central purpose may be collected in the vicinity of the operation itself.

2. The factors which determine the duration of sampling or the volume of the air to be sampled are as follows:
   a. Sensitivity of the analytical procedure
   b. The threshold limit value (TLV) of the particular contaminant
   c. The expected air concentration.

   Another considerable necessity in determining the duration of the sampling is that it should usually represent a complete cycle of operations. This is useful in determining the operator's weighted exposure. Another technique is to sample on a regular schedule, e.g. so many minutes every hour. This procedure usually requires collection of a greater number of samples than cyclic sampling procedure and is more or less substituting statistical approach for observation.
3. The number of samples to be collected depends on the purpose of sampling. The efficiency of the control measures method is in operation and the other while it is switched off. On the other hand, large number of samples may be necessary to accurately define average daily exposure for a worker engaged in the particular operation; the concentration of the airborne contaminant is also a factor to determine the number of samples needed. A few samples may be sufficient of the concentration if definitely high but if it is near TLV, a minimum of 3–5 samples may be necessary to indicate exposure for a certain task of cycle of operation.

Sampling Instruments

The basic requirements of any air sampling instruments are:

a. Source of suction, which may be an electrically or hand operated pump, an aspirator or squeeze bulb.
b. Collecting medium: It should be able to efficiently retain the contaminants to be sampled by absorption, an aspirator or mechanical retention and control.
c. Flowmeter to indicate and control the rate of suction of air to calculate the amount of air sampled. The flowmeter attached to instrument must be calibrated with wet or dry meter.

Sampling and Analysis of Gases and Vapors

Sampling Method

The two basic methods employed to collect the gaseous contaminants:

1. Use a gas collector, such as an evacuated flask. The collector is resealed immediately to prevent loss before the sample is analysed.
2. Passing a known volume of gas or air through an absorbing medium to remove the desired contaminants from the sampled atmosphere. The absorbing medium is chosen according to its efficiency for a particular contaminant.

Gas collector sample may be used to determine composition of the atmosphere to a specific time. However, the later device, i.e. passing air through an absorbing medium should be adopted for collecting continuous samples of a non-uniform atmosphere so that the average composition during a period of time can be estimated.

Sampling for the Particulates

The particulates are classified according to their physical state, i.e. liquid and solid. Liquid particles are usually classified as mists, but if the size is smaller, they are termed as fog. Solid are categorized as dust, fumes and smokes. Dust is formed through some mechanical process such as crushing, drilling and grinding. Fumes reformed by combustion sublimation or condensation processes and term is generally applied to metal oxides of zinc, magnesium, iron, lead and others. Smoke is generated as a result of combustion of organic material.

Usual sizes of contaminants	
Gases and vapors	0.0005–0.01 μ
Mists	50–100 μ
Fogs	1–50 μ
Fumes	0.001–100 μ
Dusts	0.1–1000 μ
Smokes	0.01–1 μ

These particulate exhibits similar behavior when airborne. There are various methods suggested for collecting the particulates including settling scrubbing, filtration, impingement, Tyndal effect, electrostatic precipitations, thermal precipitation and recently the photometric methods.

Respirable Dust Sampling

The US Atomic Energy Commission has defined the respirable fraction of dust in term of sampling efficiency curve which passes through the following points.

100% efficiency at 2 μ

50% efficiency at 2.5 μ

0% efficiency at 10 μ

Other criteria for the respirable fraction of dust adopted by Johannesburg Pneumoconiosis Conference (1959) are defined by a sampling efficiency curve which passes through the following points.

100% efficiency at 1 μ

50% efficiency at 5 μ

0% efficiency at 7 μ

As per (Indian) Factories Act, 1948:

Fraction passing a size-selector with the following characteristics	
Aerodynamic diameter (μm) (unit density sphere)	*% passing selector*
≤2	90
2.5	75
3.5	50
5.0	25
10	0

The concept of the respirable fraction has been applied to the fraction of the respired that reaches in the lung and not the fraction of the airborne dust that is literally respirable. The various respirable dust sampling instruments have been developed to evaluate the industrial environment.

To get the desired respirable fraction two types of elutriators are used:

a. Horizontal elutriator
b. Cyclone elutriator.

These elutriators are connected to the dust sampling instruments to eliminate the non-respirable fraction.

Analytical Method Used for the Determination of the Contaminants

The analytical methods used to determine the concentration of the desired contaminants can be divided into two main classes—chemical and physical methods.

Chemical Methods

a. Colorimetric method: The principle of this method is the development of the color by a reagent which is indicative of the concentration of the substance to be analysed. Examples of these methods are determination of zinc, lead, mercury, etc. by dithiazone extraction.
b Ion exchange: By this technique it is possible to separate elements from one and another. Mercury in urine, fluorine in urine and flouride sample can be separated for further analysis.
c. Gravimetric method: This method depends on the formation of a precipitation or a residue which can be weighed. Example is analysis of dust samples for free silica.
d. Volumetric method: By the use of standard solution for titration. Examples are acid gases which are titrated with a basic reagent.

Physical Methods

The physical methods widely used for the determination of the various contaminants are emission spectroscopy, infrared and ultraviolet spectroscopy, infrared and ultraviolet spectroscopy, mass spectroscopy, polarography, X-ray diffraction, gas chromatograph and atomic absorption spectrophotometry.

Direct Reading Instruments for Determining Concentration of Airborne Contaminants

Colorometric Indicators

The principle of these indicators has been described earlier under colorimetric method. The three types of colorometric indicators are being used: (a) Glass indicator tubes containing solid chemicals. (b) Chemically treated filter paper. (c) Liquid reagent.

Direct Physical Method for Analysis

Number of direct reading instruments has been developed by various manufacturing organisations based on the physical method for analysis. The various physical method applied have already been briefed earlier.

The factors taken into consideration for selecting particular instrument are simplicity, specificity, stability and accuracy.

THRESHOLD LIMIT VALUES

Threshold limit values (TLVs) for chemical substances in workroom air adopted by American Conference of Governmental Industrial Hygienists (ACGIH) refers to airborne concentration of substances which believed to have no adverse effect on the health or comfort of the workers repeatedly exposed day after day.

TLV Concept

The concept of the use of the exposure limits as a mean of protecting workers' health has evolved from the industrial hygiene community in developing and using such limit. One of the major contributing factors toward occupational health hazard is the prevalence of the toxic airborne contaminants in workroom air. Although all chemical substances are toxic at some concentration, a concentration exists for all substances from which no injurious effect will result, no matter how often the exposure is repeated. This concentration has been termed threshold limit value (TLV), for the substance present in the workroom air. This value is taken as guideline to control the exposure to the toxic airborne substances encountered in an industrial environment. The best practice is to maintain concentrations of all contaminants as low as possible, ideally a zero level, by applying engineering and other control methods. But in many industrial situations the achievement of the zero level of the contaminants in the workroom air is uneconomical, inapplicable or impracticable. Hence the TLVs serve as a practicable guideline to control the airborne contaminants in an industrial environment. For those substances which are absorbed through skin, mere air monitoring is not sufficed as this does not account for the dermal exposure. In such cases the total exposure through all the routes of entries (inhalation, dermal and oral) is evaluated by biochemical monitoring, i.e. by determining the urinary or blood levels of the toxic substances under investigation or its metabolite. Hence the concept of the Biological Threshold Limit Values (BTLVs) has been brought forward in the recent years. Currently the BTLV for some of the toxic substances have been recommended. With a view towards this concept of TLV or BTLV, industrial hygiene studies are conducted.

Categorization of TLVs

The TLVs currently have been categorized as follows:

1. Threshold limit value: Long-term exposure limit (LTEL), time weighted average (TLV-TWA)—The time weighted average concentration for a normal 8 hours workday to which nearly all may be repeatedly exposed without adverse effect.
2. Threshold limit value: Short-term exposure limit (TLV-STEL)—The maximal concentration to which worker can be exposed for a period of 15 minutes continuously without suffering from (1) irritation (2) chronic or irreversible change (3) narcosis of sufficient degree to increase accident proneness, impair self-rescue, or materially reduce work efficiency, provided no >4 excursions per day are permitted with at least 60 minutes between exposure period and provided that the daily TLV-TWA is also not exceeded.
3. Threshold limit value-ceiling (TLV-C): The concentration that should not be exceeded during any part of the working exposure.

Threshold limit values are based on the best available information from industrial experience from experimental human and animal studies and if possible, combination of the three TLVs are reviewed and revised every year where necessary. The guiding factors to decide a TLV may differ from substance to substance. In some cases, the impairment of health may be a guideline whereas reasonable freedom from irritation, narcosis, nuisance or other form of information available for establishing a TLV varies from substance to substance the latest 'Documentation of the TLV' a separate companion piece to the published TLVs may be consulted.

TLV of a Mixture

When two or more hazardous substances are present, their combined effect should be given primary consideration. In absence of information the effect of different hazards in a mixture should be considered as additive. Thus, if the sum of the following fraction, $C_1/T_1 + C_2/T_2 + ... + C_n/T_n$ exceeds unit, then the TLV of the mixture should be considered a being exceeded. C_1 indicates observed airborne concentration and T_1 the corresponding TLV. Exception to above rule should be made only when there is good reason to believe that the hazards of the components of mixture are not additives.

In a special case when source of contaminant is a liquid mixture and the atmospheric composition is assumed to be similar to that of the original material the TLV of the mixture (in mg/m^3) is computed by the formula:

$$\text{TLV (mixture)} = \frac{1}{\text{Fa/TLVa} + \text{Fb/TLVb} + \text{Fc/TLVc} + \text{Fn/TLVn}}$$

where, F is the fractional concentration of solvents of the mixture.

In the TLV-booklet the substances listed with 'skin' notation refers to chemical which absorbed through skin and eye also. Hence appropriate measures for prevention of cutaneous (skin) absorption should be taken so that the threshold limit value is not invalidated as this for inhalation route of entry.

Carcinogens with no Assigned TLV

For the human carcinogens, viz. chloromethyl methyl ether, 4-aminodiphenyl (p-xenylamine) benzidine, 4-nitrodiphenyl, acrylonitrite and 1,2-dibromoethene (ethylene dibromide) no TLV has been assigned. For these substances no exposure or any route, i.e. respiratory, skin or as detected by the most sensitive methods are permitted. No exposure or contact means hermitizing the process or operation by best practicable engineering methods. The worker should be properly equipped to ensure virtually no contact with the carcinogens.

Biological Monitoring

Biologic monitoring was defined by a seminar sponsored by the European Economic Community (EEC), the National Institute for Occupational Safety and Health (NIOSH) and Occupational Safety and Health Administration (OSHA) as "the measurement and assessment of agents or their metabolites either in tissues, secreta, excreta, expired air or any combination of these to evaluate exposure and health risk, compared to an appropriate reference". Unlike air or surface monitoring which assess potential exposure, biological monitoring can help to assess actual systemic exposure, from all routes. BM is particularly useful where air monitoring alone will not give a complete picture of exposure. In most countries, there is a legal requirement for health surveillance of workers who may be significantly exposed to chemical, e.g. lead.

A relatively new approach to worker protection is to introduce individualized tests that measure exposure rather than clinical impairment or abnormality. Biological monitoring is a technology based on toxicology that is designed to evaluate individual exposure. Biological monitoring is a very precise term for the periodic evaluation of the workers by detecting the indicators of exposure through trace residues of the agent, its metabolites, or a biological response. These methods are designed to quantify levels of internal dose following exposures lower than would be implicated as a cause of illness. For example, the free erythrocytic protoporphyrin assay on blood detects exposure to lead at levels far below that required to cause illness and is more reliable an indicator of body burden than blood lead levels. End-expired breath carbon monoxide levels give a very precise indication of exposure to carbon monoxide during a shift. Likewise, end-expired breath solvent measured by mass spectroscopy gives a very accurate picture of the individual exposure to these agents, as levels far below the current threshold limit values (TLVs). Biological monitoring will proceed by the establishment of biologic exposure indices (BEIs). This represents a substantial step forward in monitoring technology.

Biological monitoring (BM) is based on the analysis of hazardous substances or their metabolites in biological fluids, usually urine, blood or breath. BM is a tool to assess systemic exposure and reflect absorption by all routes: inhalation, ingestion and through the skin. Often, the term 'biological monitoring' is also used to include biological effect monitoring (BEM), which reflect the early consequences of systemic exposure, although others have also used the term 'biomonitoring' to encompass BM and BEM. Both BM and BEM are located on a spectrum ranging from low exposure at one end to disease, frank toxicity or death at the other end. It is preferable to keep the term 'biological monitoring' for assessment of exposure separate from 'biological effect monitoring' which is an indicator of early effect and sits within 'health surveillance'. Health surveillance is the periodic clinical examination of workers designed to protect their health through the early detection of adverse effects and intervention to prevent further harm, and complements biological monitoring. Monitoring techniques can be divided into those that assess exposure and those that assess the consequences of exposure. Thus, BM relates to exposure assessment and BEM is usually part of effects assessment, and can help in the diagnosis of disease.

Principal Biological Monitoring Methods

The biological monitoring of exposure is based on the determination of indicators of internal dose by measuring:

1. The amount of the chemical, to which the worker is exposed, in blood or urine (rarely in milk, saliva, or fat).
2. The amount of one or more metabolites of the chemical involved in the same body fluids.
3. The concentration of volatile organic compounds (solvents) in alveolar air.
4. The biological effective dose of compounds which have formed adducts to DNA or other large molecules and which thus have a potential genotoxic effect.

Biological effect monitoring, susceptibility and diagnosis: There are some areas of uncertainty about where some analysis may be better considered as biological monitoring, biological effect monitoring or better defined as diagnosis of overt occupational disease. For example, blood carboxyhemoglobin (COHb) could be considered a classical BEM marker for situation where there is direct exposure to carbon monoxide, from an industrial process, and through the metabolism of dichloromethane and smoking status. Circulating levels of COHb are both a direct indicator of the reduced oxygen-carrying capacity of blood and an indirect marker of likely tissue anoxia. The relationship between COHb and the classical toxic symptoms are well-defined, so that health-based occupational limits have been readily set. Breath carbon monoxide is a non-invasive measurement that can be assessed on site using readily available instrument and showing a good relationship with COHb levels. Thus, in this case, the distinction between BM and BEM is arbitrary, and in higher exposures COHb is the diagnostic test confirming possible symptoms of frank toxicity and the possible need for the aggressive therapy, such as hyperbaric oxygen.

RISK MANAGEMENT AT WORKPLACE

In occupational medicine, three applications of the scientific aspects of toxicology are particularly important, they are: risk assessment, individual variation in clinical toxicology, and biological monitoring.

Risk Assessment

Hazard control and prevention in the workplace depend on toxicology to establish the relationship between levels of exposure and potential risk for a member of the exposed group. To be of use of setting standards and evaluating policy alternatives, the findings of occupational epidemiology studies must be relevant to human health effects likely to occur. Risk assessment is a process of estimating the probability of harm or damage occurring within a population as a result of a particular hazard, a means of introducing rigor into the evaluation of a possible threat to health. Risk assessment uses the technique of toxicology and epidemiology to assess the hazard posed by the substance, its risk to those exposed, and the trade-offs implicit in setting standards and public policy to protect those who may be exposed. A typical risk assessment exercise begins by defining the level of hazard posed by a particular exposure, normally in the form of an exposure-response relationship.

Individual Factors in Clinical Toxicology

The mechanism of biological variation is fundamental to understand exposure related outcomes because it is these mechanisms that oppose the action of the toxic result. The efficient interpretation of population data to yield clues to the mechanism of toxicity depends on the knowledge of the biologic mechanisms of xenobiotic metabolism and host defense mechanisms.

Biological Monitoring

Biological monitoring is a technology based on toxicology that is designed to evaluate individual exposure. Biological monitoring is a very precise term for the periodic evaluation of the workers by detecting the indicators of exposure through trace residues of the agent, its metabolites, or a biological response.

Environmental Risk Assessment Process

The policies and laws that are written to address concerns about environmental pollution, occupational hazards, and the protection of human health usually rely on information taken from a myriad of sources, some of that are process-based, and some are value-based or based on the systematic analysis. Therefore, a *risk assessment* methodology has been developed and applied to evaluate the impact the pollution on the environment and ecosystems and, to a lesser degree, on quality-of-life issues. Risk can be defined as the probability or chance that an unwanted action, circumstances, or event will result in loss or harm. Risk assessment is a means or methodology to quantify risk, but it is important to recognize that it is a process. The process of risk assessment uses scientific data, statistical and mathematical methodology, and expert judgment to characterize the probability for an adverse outcome. In its most basic form, risk assessment is the process through which toxicology data collected from animal studies and human exposure studies are combined with information about the degree of exposure to predict the likelihood that a particular adverse response will be seen in the individual or the population.

The US National Research Council defines risk assessment as a four-step process developed to aid in the evaluation of the safety of systematic chemical use or the exposure of human from chemicals in the environment (Fig. 2.4). The four steps of risk assessment are:

1. *Hazard identification*: Hazard identification is the step in which it is determined whether exposure to an agent could cause an increase in the incidence of adverse health effects in humans. It is the qualitative evaluation of the adverse health effect of a substance. Many factors are considered in this determination, and depending on the toxicological endpoint of concern, there might be specific additional factors to consider.
2. *Dose-response assessment*: Dose-response evaluations define the relationship between the dose of an agent and the observance or expected occurrence of a specific toxicological effect in the environment or workplace. It is a process of estimating the relation between the dose of a substance and the incidence of an adverse health effect.
3. *Exposure assessment*: The elimination of the exposure of a toxic substance would result in zero risk. Because the total elimination of chemical exposure often is not feasible or practical, the exposure assessment step in a risk assessment is used to estimate the magnitude and probability of uptake from the environment by any combination of oral, inhalation, and dermal route of exposure. The results of the exposure assessment are quantitative doses presented in the amount of the chemical per unit of body weight per unit of time (e.g. mg/kg per day).
4. *Risk characterization*: In the risk characterization, it is required to summarize and interpret the information collected from the previous three steps, presents a quantitative estimate of the human health risks, and identifies the uncertainties in these risk estimates. This process allows identifying the greatest individual and population health risks and promulgating health-based action levels to protect individuals and populations from further exposure or to prevent immediate or long-term injury. It is the process of estimating the probable incidence of an adverse health effect to human under various conditions of exposure, including a description of the uncertainties involve. It is dependent on information derived from exposure and dose-response assessment, and

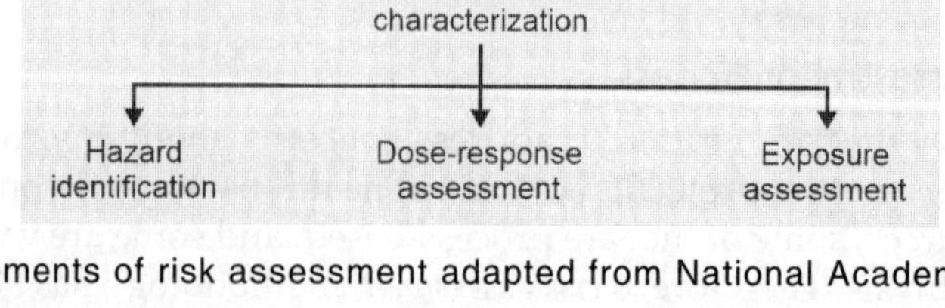

Fig. 2.4: Elements of risk assessment adapted from National Academy of Science

these three elements combined are often referred to as quantitative risk assessment (QRA). The hazards identification element has also been frequently referred to as quantitative risk assessment.

The second process is called *risk management,* and it uses a value-based approach to determine what level of risk to human health will be considered significant and to formulate options for identifying, selecting, and implementing action to prevent, reduce, or maintain risks below that level. Risk management considers risk along with other technical, economic, legal, and social factors. The third element of the risk assessment model, *risk communication,* was added later with the intent of linking risk assessors with the public by presenting information in the most effective way.

ACUTE VS CHRONIC OCCUPATIONAL HEALTH EFFECTS

- A chronic health effect is an adverse health effect resulting from long-term exposure to a substance, e.g. silicosis, asbestosis, etc.
- Acute health effects can be observed immediately or soon after an exposure; often a large, brief exposure, e.g. irritant effects of chlorine, ammonia, etc.

METHOD OF CONTROLLING AIRBORNE CONTAMINANTS

Airborne contaminants may be in the form of dusts, fumes, vapors, gases and mists. The contaminants arise in industry in many ways like:

1. Raw materials for the process itself may be hazardous—silica, chlorine.
2. Contamination may be due to the nature of the finished product like manufacture of CO.
3. Contamination may be due to breakdown in the plant or the control measure employed to prevent the contaminant escaping into the atmosphere.
4. Contamination may be due to release of toxic materials ancillary to the product like dust generated in weaving asbestos, contamination of atmosphere from 'spotting' in garment cleaning industry.
5. Airborne poisons may also arise incidentally to the handling or transport of materials even in the course of manufacture either in raw state or as finished products.

The greatest danger from airborne contaminants is due to their entry into the body through the lungs, but atmospheric contamination is harmful in other ways also like dermatitis, skin cancer (if the atmosphere contains carcinogens).

Apart from the principles of prevention which will be dealt with later there are certain basic requirements which are necessary. The structure of the building should be sound and suited to its process. Drainage, water, supply, sanitation and high standard of housekeeping and disposal of rubbish and sweeping and washing of floors, etc. are a few to be mentioned. These requirements are basic of healthy conditions everywhere but assume great importance where poisonous materials are used.

Principles of Prevention

1. Substitution
2. Segregation
3. Enclosures

4. Exhaust ventilation
5. General ventilation
6. Wet methods
7. Personal protection
8. Warning and publicity.

This is more or less the order of importance of these principles and applying them to any particular hazard should always be sought by the use of a method of prevention higher on the list in preference to which is lower. For example, substitution should be attempted before exhaust ventilation is considered and exhaust ventilation should be applied before wet methods or personal protection or worker is contemplated. It is possible to ensure maximum protection if this method is followed. It will be noticed that there is bound to be some over lapping in the control measures. For instance, segregation may involve some type of enclosure and exhaust ventilation may involve both.

Substitution

This is the most effective method of controlling an industrial toxic hazard but it is by no means very popular. The reason is that a change in material in an industrial process is fundamental and when this is asked for only on the grounds not connected with the efficiency of the plant, the management is reluctant to do it. A change is also resisted by the employees who are used to old habits and ways of working as well as by the consumers who may be prejudiced against change in the product which may affect the soiling points, e.g. domestic cleaning powders may contain high percentage of silica flour and pumica is a satisfactory substitute but is darker in colour and generally a white powder would be pre-ferred to a grey powder for cleaning. Cost may be another factor in preventing the use of safe material instead of unsafe material. If the cost difference is very high only some sort of legislation may have to be applied to induce the manufacturers in not using dangerous materials. But if such legislation does not exist all over the world it may result in loss of market to countries that are progressing in their attitude in industrial poisons.

Perhaps one of the earliest legislations was requiring the use of red phosphorus instead of white phosphorus. In some countries there is prohibition in the use of (a) Sandblasting; (b) Use of low flush point solvents in dry cleaning; (c) Use of CS_2 in Rubber Industry; (d) Use of raw lead glazes in pottery industry.

Segregation

The principle is to confine the danger to few persons.

a. Distance: Keeping the dangerous materials away from other parts of the works. This may limit the exposure to a few persons or to exclude it entirely. Distance is the simplest, cheapest and safest means of protection against a wide range of radioactive exposures.
b. Distance in conjunction with enclosure or other protective arrangement.
c. Segregation without distances: Part of the plant may be separated from the rest by partition of the premises. Segregation has many advantages where; the risk of poisoning is not mainly from airborne contaminants. It helps to prevent contamination being carried elsewhere.
d. Segregation of the process from particular classes of persons, e.g. prohibition of employment of women and young persons where lead is handled as they are more susceptible to lead poisoning.

Enclosure

Segregation and enclosures are generally considered together. Enclosure means some physical separation of toxic material or processes from the workroom in such a way as to prevent any contamination of the surroundings and this principle of control should always be considered before. Elaborate and expensive ventilation systems are proposed. Also designing of a ventilation system becomes much easier and less costly if, the contaminants are contained in a small space. In some industries, enclosure is necessary for the process itself like oil refining, tar distillation and many chemical processes which are continuous or semicontinuous and the plant has to be completely closed to the atmosphere for cost consideration and to prevent evaporation losses. Similarly, enclosure is necessary where solvents and other volatile substances are used and atmospheric contamination is also prevented. Most of the accidents in enclosed plants occur due to inadequate maintenance which may lead to unexpected leakage, or when going into vessels and other confined spaces for repairs and maintenance. 'Permit to work' system and regular sampling around the plant is necessary to detect escape of contaminants. Besides the industries where it is necessary to enclose the plant, enclosure can be adopted as a precaution in processes for prevention of escape of contaminants. Section 14 of the Factories Act and Rules framed under Section 87 of the Act require certain controls to be provided in certain dangerous operations to prevent the escape of dust and fumes. It is obligatory 'on the part of the management' to provide this enclosure in such cases is a very useful and practical means of control, e.g. (a) Treatment of cloth where materials or solvents are used. (b) Processes involving use of Formaldehyde. (c) Handling or bagging of powders can be completely enclosed.

Local Exhaust and General Ventilation

Though some of the problems of pollution of working environment can be tackled by making slight changes in the raw materials or operation, if it be possible without determinant to the process, yet one single method which is applicable to most of the problems is ventilation. General or dilution ventilation is not recommended for toxic contaminants. Dilution by natural air currents or by mechanic means like exhaust fan is applied only in the case of low toxicity solvents and alcohols, otherwise, extraction of contaminants at the source by local exhaust ventilation is the only dependable solution. Operations should be maximally enclosed. Minimum required openings of the operations should be locally exhausted. Various types of exhaust hoods and slots have been devised for different operation.

Wet Methods

Use of water to prevent the escape of dust into the atmosphere is an age-old method. It is cheap and simple but it can be fully effective only in a limited number of applications. The main applications may be:

a. As a direct method of controlling dust by spray or other means.
b. As a method of preventing dust arising by handling materials in a wetted state.
c. As an ancillary precaution where other measure relied upon as a main precaution. In some countries wet methods are required to be used by law.

Dust Suppression

Jets or sprays applied to cutting tools chisels, saws in the cutting or handling of stone, etc. grinding of metals by grinding wheels. In the suppression of dust by wetting now dry surface is continuously formed and wetting of smallest dust particles is difficult and dust levels below permissible levels may not be assured. In case of water sprays, water wets the whole of the surroundings and thus prevents emission of dust. The actual quantity of water used is important.

Dust Prevention

Dust prevention by wet methods is more successful than dust suppression. Adequate supplies of water and time factor are important. Material that has been wetted must not be allowed to dry nut again. This also creates problems for disposal of sludge formed in wetting process. Handling of materials in paste form instead of as a powder is another method, e.g. (a) Application of talc in rubber industry, by dipping the material in water suspension of talc. (b) Wet abrasives used for cleaning castings.

Use of Personal Protective Equipment

A. Respiratory: For gases, etc.
   a. Chemical cartridge respirator.
   b. Canister gas masks.
   c. Self-contained breathing apparatus (oxygen or air).
   d. Supplied air breathing apparatus. For dust: Mechanical filters (ordinary and micro-filters).

B. Non-respiratory: Gloves, aprons, overalls, goggles, face shield, foot and leg protection.

Personal Cleanliness

Wash-ups, bathing facilities, cloak rooms to discard work clothes and to keep other clothing.

Medical Examination

Pre-employment and periodical medical examination.

Education and Training of Workers

Education and Training of Workers on Personal Hygiene

Health Awareness Program to develop positive knowledge, attitude and practice (KAP) of the workers in the industry should be conducted regularly for the promotion and maintenance of the highest degree of physical, mental and social well-being of the workers of the factory. Improvement of environmental health is a major concern of many industries. The objectives of health education in environmental health promotion through improvement of personal hygiene are:

1. To educate the people in the principle of environmental health with a view to bring about desired changes in health practice.
2. To secure adoption, wide use and maintenance of environmental health practice.
3. To promote active participation of the people to improve the personal and environmental health.

Chapter

3

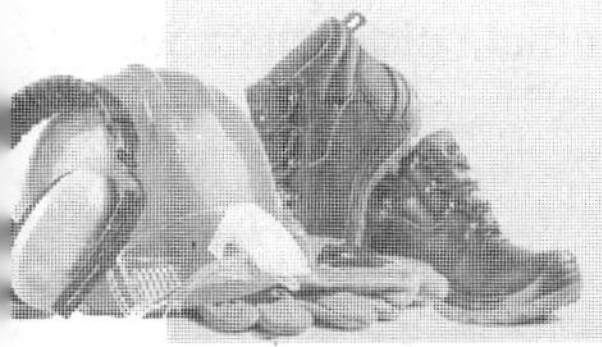

Industrial Physiology

Industrial/work physiology is the discipline that analyses the responses of the human organism to physical activity and to the different stresses occurring during work. It measures the physiological cost of different work methods to determine how work should be performed with the least energy expenditure and with least fatigue. Ergonomic is concerned with the knowledge from basic science such as 'physiology', 'anatomy' and 'psychology'. *Environmental physiology* is the study of interaction of the living organism with physical factors of the environment, such as climate, noise and vibration, light, gaseous composition of air. *Engineering psychology* is the discipline that studies the sensory and mental capacities of man in order to establish the conditions under which a man-machine system can most efficiently and safely operate. It also deals with the behavioral factors of performance and fatigue, such as motivation, vigilance, information proceeding, decision-making and learning. Other important areas are the interaction between physical and mental work and the effect of environmental factors on human proficiency. The expression 'environmental factor' is used here in the broadest sense, and environment refers to both physical and psychosocial environments.

Before individual workers are allotted industrial jobs, and often subsequently as well, it is necessary that their physical abilities are measured against the jobs which they will be required to performed. Such assessment may require the application of techniques, the use of which does not obtain in the routine methodology of clinical examination. The choice of the method, or methods, of assessment depends on the nature of the job to be performed by the workers. Fitness presents a dual face, one side reflects the functional and anatomical endowment of the subject examined, the other the task to which the individual is operationally fitted. Fitness and its reciprocal, unfitness, the latter intended as a medical statement of real limits, are complex entities based on the functional, anatomic, psychologic, educational and social characteristics of the workers, since all these factors interact with the mechanical and dynamic demands of a job performance. It is precisely this relational characteristic of matching a person to a given task that is the essence of the fitness assessment process.

The whole process of determining fitness is a series of measurement and as such, is an exercise in relativity. The extent of fitness or impairment must be gauged in terms of the demand of the task to be performed, specified in type, intensity, duration and schedule. Appropriate considerations for the specific task for which the fitness evaluation is requested, inclusive of the environment and the structure in which the job takes place, e.g. ambient physical factors, work schedule, work-pause sequence, technology, etc. are important.

More sophisticate items of equipment used to test work capacity include mechanically or electrically braked ergometers and variable-inclined treadmills (Fig. 3.1). With these devices, a subject is tested at progressively higher loads (stepwise), each applied for a duration between 1 and 5 minutes. The heart rate is monitored which increases in linear, in correspondence to increased loads, the extrapolation to maximal load can be obtained from submaximal task. In addition to heart rate, subjective perception of tolerance, i.e. fatigue should be obtained to define better maximal limits. The continuous electrocardiographic (ECG) monitoring makes the assessment more informative. However, it should be remembered that minor abnormalities in ECG records may be noted during exercise in 75% of male and 50% of female older than 50 years of age, suggesting a generally benign nature of these findings (Fig. 3.2).

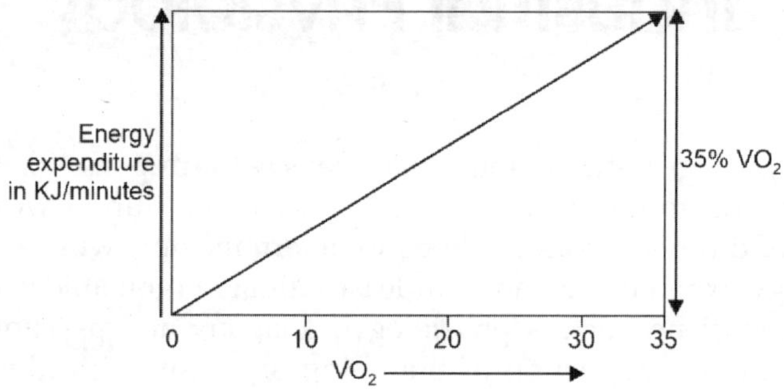

Fig. 3.1: Volume of O_2 vs energy consumption

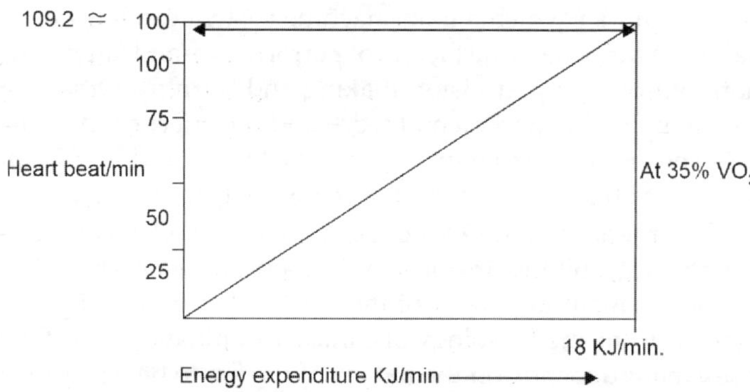

Fig. 3.2: Heart beat vs energy expenditure

CLASSIFICATION OF WORKLOAD—WORK CAPACITY AND MAN-JOB ALIGNMENT

Acceptable Workload for Indian Workers

An acceptable workload for Indian worker may be defined that workload which can be performed in 8 hours without fatigue by a worker. One hour lunch and 15 minutes tea break in two halves of shift are considered to calculate acceptable workload (Fig. 3.3).

Method of Determination of Rest Periods and Acceptable Workload

What do you understand by physiological classification of workload? Mention about the components of physiological parameters by which workload in industry can be classified:

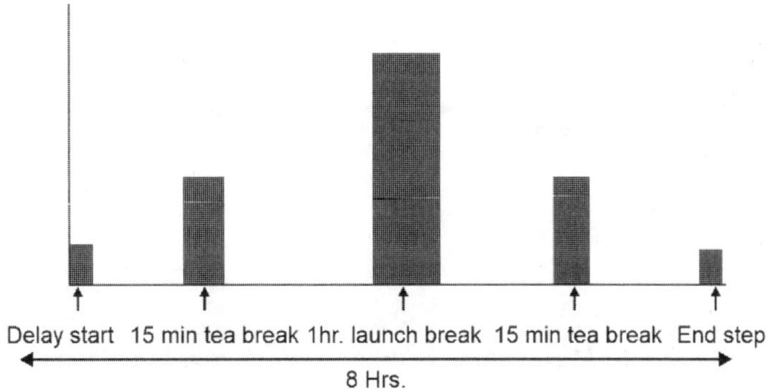

Fig. 3.3: Acceptable workload

Physiological classification of workload summarises some of the physiological variables. Physiological variables or measurements are the heart beat rate, the oxygen consumption, the sweating rate, energy expenditure and oral temperature.

The workload is classified into five types, i.e. light, moderate, heavy, very heavy and unduly work. The important of classification of workload is to:

1. Know the severity of worker's condition.
2. Know energy expenditure.
3. Right person to right job.

Workload classification

Physiological variables	*Light work*	*Moderate work*	*Heavy work*	*Very work*	*Unduly work*	*Reference*
Energy expenditure (KJ/min)	1–2.5	2.5–4.00	4–6	6–8	>8.0	Ramanathan and Dutta (1967), JIAOH, Bombay
Pulse rate (beat/min)	75–100	100–125	125–150	150–175	>175	Christensen (1963), 'Men at work'
Oral temp °C (not <3 min)	Normal	36.9–37.4	37.4–37.9	37.9–38.4	>38.4	do
Sweating rate ml/hr. (average for 8 hr. work)	Normal	200–400	400–600	600–800	>800	do

VO_2 Max

A more realistic and informative assessment of the physiologic cost of mechanical work is obtained with the measure of oxygen consumption (VO_2). When this measurement is obtained at maximum workload, it is called maximum aerobic capacity of VO_2 max. Aerobic capacity and mechanical workload is directly related through the efficiency factor, based on VO_2, measured for its ability to assess mechanical work. Since any muscular work operates on oxidative processes, the oxygen consumed during a given activity directly quantifies the muscular work done. Different mechanical operations can, therefore, be estimated through VO_2 by the simple device of monitoring oxygen ($VO_2 = VO_2$ inspired – VO_2 expired). After a particular level of work, if the work is increased, the Vo_2 will not increase and the linear presentation will show a platue after VO_2 max (Fig. 3.4a and b).

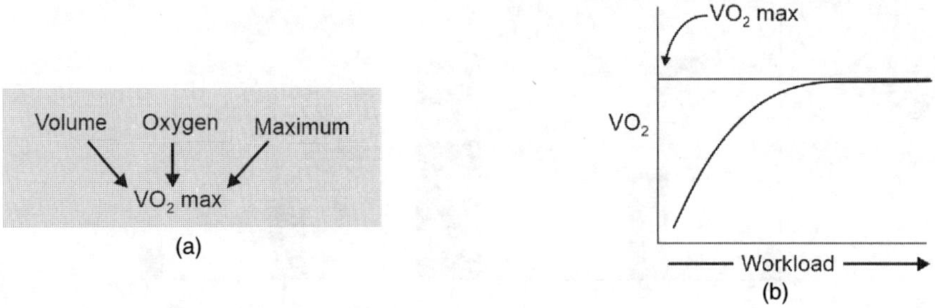

Fig. 3.4a and b: Maximum volume of oxygen your body can utilize

FATIGUE

Fatigue can be described as a state which is characterized by a feeling of tiredness combined with a reduction or undesired variation in the performance of the activity. It is found that after fairly prolonged heavy work there is a reduction of capacity, i.e. usually called *fatigue*. This does not apply to muscular activity alone. The sensory organs or the nerve centers are also become tired. It is, however, the aim of every cell to balance out the capacity lost by its activity, a process which is called *recovery*. The concepts of fatigue and recovery at human work are closely related to the ergonomic concepts of stress and strain. Stress means the sum of all parameters of work in the working system influencing people at work, which are perceived or sensed mainly over the receptor system or which put demands on the effectors system.

Prolonged and strong contraction of a muscle leads to the well-known state of muscle fatigue. This results simply from inability of the contractile and metabolic processes of the muscle fibers to continue supplying the same work output. The nerve continues to function properly, the nerve impulses pass normally through the neuromuscular junction into the muscle fibers, and even normal action potentials spread over the muscle fibers, but the contraction becomes weaker and weaker because of depletion of energy supplies in the muscles fibers themselves. Interruption of blood flow through a contracting muscles lead to almost complete muscle fatigue in a minute or more because of the obvious loss of nutrient supply.

The fatigue symptoms can be divided into three categories:

1. Physiological: It results in physiological reactions like increased heart rate.
2. Behavioral: It decreases the performance parameter like increasing errors when solving certain tasks.
3. Psychophysical: It increases the feeling of exertion and deterioration.

PHYSIOLOGICAL TEST IN OCCUPATIONAL HEALTH ASSESSMENT

Harvard Step Test

The aim of Harvard Step Test is to assess the physical fitness of individuals. Fitness is defined as the job likely to be performed and the capacity to perform the job, of a person. It is the quantitative expression of the physical condition of an individual. Harvard Step Test was originally developed in Harvard Fatigue Laboratory, USA in order to determine the fitness status of an individual, especially cardiovascular fitness. This also determines the fitness to perform a specific task requiring muscular efforts in which, speed, endurance, strength and flexibility are the main criteria. Exercise involves oxygen consumption by body. Oxygen consumption or energy expenditure is directly proportional to the heart rate. Any exercise by which one reaches his maximum oxygen consumption rate is utilized for assessing the physical fitness of that individual. Harvard Step Test is one of the simplest tests to measure physical fitness. During this test an individual almost attains the maximum oxygen consumption stage. In this test the subject is asked to step up and down a 20ˆ bench/stool at a rate of 30 cycles per minutes for 5 minutes or until exhaustion, whichever is earlier. Exhaustion is defined as when the subject cannot maintain the stepping rate for 15 seconds. A 20ˆ (50.8 cm) stool or step, 2 stopwatches, a metronome (or cadence tape) and a stethoscope are required for Harvard Step Test.

Procedure

The tested subject is asked to take rest for some time before the start of the test. His resting pulse rate, height and weight are recorded. Then the subject is asked to step up and down the 20″ stool at a rate of 30 steps per minute (the rhythm is adjusted by the metronome). To complete one step, there are four sub-steps: 1st—left foot on the top of stool, 2nd—both left and right feet on the stool and stand completely on the stool, 3rd—bring right foot down on the ground and 4th—both left and right feet on ground and stand completely on the ground. The subject is advice to continue stepping for 5 minutes or until exhaustion (till he is no longer able to continue), whichever is earlier. The time taken for which the subject performs the exercise is recorded by the help of the stopwatch. As soon as the subject terminates his exercise, he is advice to sit on a nearby chair and his recovering heart rate is recorded during the period from 1 minute to 1 minute 30 seconds, 2 minutes to 2 minutes 30 seconds, and 4 minutes to 4 minutes 30 seconds with the help of stethoscope and stopwatch.

The fitness score or the physical fitness index (PFI) is calculated by using the formula:

$$\text{PFI} = \frac{\text{Duration of exercise in seconds} \times 100}{2 \times \text{Total recovering heart rate } [(1 - 1.5 \text{ min}) + (2 - 2.5 \text{ min}) + (4 + 4.5 \text{ min})]}$$

The interception of PFI is done as per the following principle:

Poor = <55 Low average = 55–64 Average = 65–79

Good = 80–90 Excellent = >90

The followings are the findings of Harvard Step Test

a. Recovering heart rate
b. Physical fitness index (PFI) in the unit of score
c. Total work done during the test and measured as:

Total work done
= Body weight in kg × height of stool in mtr. × cycle per minute × duration of test in min.
= kg × (51/100) × 30 × duration of test in minute.

In Harvard Step Test, height of stool and cycle per minute are fixed, i.e. {(51/100)m × 30/m}. The body weight of the subject and his duration of performance are variable.

ERGONOMICS

Ergonomics may be defined as the science of 'man at work'—fitting the job to the man. It is concerned with the knowledge from basic science such as 'Physiology', 'Anatomy' and

'Psychology' about limitations and capabilities of human-beings and integrating this knowledge with information from applied studies such as engineering and management studies in the interest of matching task demands with human limitations. This knowledge can be applied in the work sites to achieve the highest standard of reciprocal adaptation between man and his work—both humanitarian and economic ends. In 1961, the International Labour Review defined ergonomics as "the application of the human biological sciences in conjunction with the engineering sciences to achieve the optimum mutual adjustment of man and his work, the benefits being measured in terms of human efficiency and well-being". This mutual adaptation reduces stress, lightens the workload and increases safety; equipment and plant are used more efficiently, and their reliability is improved.

It is now a well-recognized discipline and constitutes an integral part of any advanced occupational health service. The term 'ergonomics' is derived from the Greek words 'ergon' meaning 'work' and 'nomos' meaning 'law'. Training in ergonomics involves designing of machine, tools, equipment and manufacturing process, layout of the places of work, methods of work and environment in order to achieve greater efficiency of both man and machine. The objective of ergonomics is 'to achieve the best mutual adjustment of man and his work, for the improvement of the human efficiency and well-being'. The application of ergonomics has made a significant contribution to reduce industrial accidents and to the overall health and efficiency of the workers. The causative factors for ergonomic hazards include improperly designed tools, equipment or work areas; unusual and unnecessary lifting or reaching; poor visual conditions; excessive vibration; or repeated forceful motions in awkward postures. These factors may be responsible for fatigue, stress, and strain, as well as cumulative trauma disorders and other musculoskeletal injuries. They may also predispose workers to harm from other safety hazards.

Ergonomics may be considered as the meeting point of variety of disciplines such as 'anthropometry and biomechanics', 'occupational physiology (work physiology and environmental physiology)'. 'Occupational health', 'work planning', 'operational research', 'engineering psychology' and 'cybernetics (the science of communications and control in machines, e.g. computers and living things)". The study in individual problems and the overall analysis of specific situations contributed to the enlargement of knowledge in each discipline; however, it is primarily in the design of improved work posts, methods and equipment that ergonomics makes itself felt as an independent and integrated discipline. This necessitates collaboration between the 'research worker' and the technician, and specialist use of observation, measurement, recording and testing equipment. Thus, the ergonomist forms part of a multidisciplinary ergonomic-team.

Anthropometry and biomechanics are the disciplines that establish the principles and standards for the design of equipment, workplace and motion pattern for different operations to bring them into harmony with the size, shape, mobility and structure of the human body. The aim is to enable a man to exert the greatest force with highest precision speed and safety and with the least-effort.

Application of Ergonomics

Ergonomics can be applied to any activity where human effort is involved—at home, in offices, factories and workhouses—on the seas, in the air, and even in spaces. Thus, it has been successfully applied in:

1. Design of furniture, seats, rests and steps for operators.
2. Design of jigs and fixtures.

3. Improvement in working conditions and environments.
4. Selection, training and placement of personnel.
5. Motivation of workers.
6. Fatigue reduction.
7. Betterment of health and safety standards.
8. Composition of 'relaxation allowances' for workers, etc.

Anthropometric data—height, length of arms and of legs and many others are needed to fit the machine to the man. A study of loads—physical, perceptual and mental–static and dynamic posture, pauses of rest–tend to better understanding of problems of performance and contribute more comfort, less fatigue and better productivity. Similarly, hours of work, temperature, humidity, illumination, noise, altitude—each plays its role and better understanding of their role leads to more ease, more comfort and more work. Contrary to popular beliefs, more hours of work do not mean more overall production. A reduction in the number of hours worked per week has been found to produce an increase in the rate of production in case of heavy work. This effect however, is not so pronounced in the case of light work.

Ergonomics and Biomechanics

An important field for the ergonomist is locomotion and posture that involve both energy expenditure and the sensorimotor features. Here he can have recourse to biomechanics. When dealing with the fit worker he must ensure that the postural stresses are reduced, training is given in kinetic methods and manual handling, seats in the plant and on vehicles are comfortable, levers, pedals and other controls are accessible and that the worker receives adequate physical training either in his work or by some sporting activity; in the case of the handicapped, thought should be given to rehabilitation, the supply of prostheses and specialized equipment.

ANTHROPOMETRY

Anthropometry is a fundamental branch of physical anthropology. It represents the quantitative aspect. A wide system of theories and practice is devoted to defining methods and variables to relate the aims in the different fields of application. In the fields of occupational health, safety and ergonomics anthropometric systems are mainly concerned with body build, composition and constitution, and with the dimensions of the human body's interrelation to workplace dimensions machines, the industrial environment and clothing.

ADAPTING MAN TO HIS WORK

Although it is essential to adapt the work to the man, ergonomics can also help adapt man to his job. The psychologist and industrial sociologist have gone into these matters thoroughly. The ergonomist can help here by his knowledge of training problems and suggesting teaching moods; this he will do in the light of cybernetic theory, his proposals relating to such things as apprenticeship programs, programming and teaching aids. Clearly, the understanding as well as the worker will derive benefit from this. Applied psychology will be used to assist in the choice and training of persons whose jobs necessitate an ability to handle large amount of information, reach quickly or cope with an emergency. A study of social factors and their effects on worker's outlook is also of value and should cover attitudes, motives and human relations and communications between workers and with other people. Acclimatization is basically one of the adaptation principles of working in heat prone areas.

SUSTAIN TRAUMA INJURY (STI)/CUMULATIVE TRAUMA DISORDERS

Musculoskeletal disorders (MSDs) rank first in frequency among work-related injuries and diseases. Musculoskeletal injuries can result from acute injuries or be chronic in nature. When related to repetitive trauma, the resulting disorders are called cumulative trauma disorders (CTDs). The human body has great recuperative powers, but when recovery time is inadequate and high repetition is combined with forceful and awkward postures, CTDs can develop. Job stress is also a factor in the multifactorial etiology model of occupationally related disorders, since psychologic stress can be associated with increase muscle tension resulting in altered muscle and tendon metabolism.

Additionally, those who treat injured workers often find poor work habits, awkward posture, aging, and inadequate self-care of the working body as a major source of CTDs in today's workers. Studies show that improving the tone of workers' musculoskeletal system with appropriate exercise reduces the incidence of worker MSDs. A job analysis system has been described that, by documenting several of the risk factors involved in CTD, enables tasks to be redesigned.

In 1986, the National Institute of Occupational Safety and Health (NIOSH) defined cumulative trauma disorders as "when job demands ... repeatedly exceed the biomechanical capacities of the worker, the activities become trauma inducing. Hence, traumatogens are workplace sources of biomechanical strain that contribute to the onset of injuries affecting the musculoskeletal systems". Thus, repeated exposure to 'traumatogens' were felt to cause accumulated injury to muscles, tendons, nerves, joints, blood vessels, or ligaments, leading to inflammation, restriction of movement, and specific disorders of these units. Cumulative trauma disorders, particularly those of the upper extremities are now widely thought to be caused, at least in part, by workplace risk factors, including awkward postures, excessive force, and repetitive movements. Research suggests a number of risk factors may foster the development of cumulative trauma disorders. Among them are:

1. Use of pinch grip.
2. Prolonged static postures.
3. Excessive bending or twisting of the wrist.
4. Continued elevation of the elbow.
5. Constant physical contact with hard work surfaces or sharp edges.
6. Temperature extremes.
7. Poorly design hand tools.
8. Inadequate space and clearances at workstations.
9. Power tool vibration.
10. Poorly designed or seating or leg support.

Undue torture to the human body or any part of the body results into various types of disorders. Excuses or improper uses of fingers lead to complaints starting from simple pain and fatigue to permanent incapability by neurological or tendon affections. Frequent movement of eyeball, leading to working of eye muscles, resulting into various eye complications. Frequent improper movement of shoulder-to-shoulder joint pains, etc. Chronic backache, a permanent feature among the industrial workers—is due to the non the non-proper support leading to muscle strain is responsible for less productivity due to chronic absenteeism and medical response. This affects them in three dimensions—economically, socially and psychologically. Naturally, the result is less output. Therefore, it is high time to care for 'man' equally if not more like 'machine', 'money' and 'material' application of human minimize the suffering of workers 'the man'.

The body parts which are most susceptible to be affected due to non or poor consideration of human factors in workplace are:

a. Upper extremity (shoulder, elbow, wrist, hand and fingers).
b. Lower extremity (knee, ankle and foot).
c. Back (spine and the muscles surrounding them).

Common Disorders of the Upper Extremity due to Improper Workplace or Tools or Work Methods

Carpal Tunnel Syndrome (CST)

CST is one of the most common and well-recognized cumulative trauma disorders of the upper extremity. It is caused by the injury to the median nerve in the wrist. The boundaries of the carpal tunnel are denoted by the carpal bones dorsally (except the pisiform) which are linked by a series of interosseous ligaments, and the transverse carpal ligament provides the origin to various thenar and hypothenar muscles. While these ligaments provide a somewhat malleable configuration of the carpal tunnel, the boundaries are rather non-yielding, a significant factor in the development of CTS. Although this tunnel run four superficial flexor tendons (the flexor digitorum superficialis), four deep flexor tendons (the flexor digitorum profundus), the flexor policis longus, and the median nerve. Conditions that increase the volume contained within the carpal tunnel, such as a swollen tendon or muscle anomaly, or decrease the area of the tunnel, as after a fracture, can increase the CT pressure and compress the only structure with elasticity within the canal—the median nerve. External compression about the wrist may also result in median nerve damage from ischemia. The median nerve supplies sensation to the palmar side of the thumb, index, middle finger, and the radial half of the ring finger. The dorsal side of these fingers distal to the proximal interphalangeal joint and the radial half of the palm are similarly innervated. Motor function of the long finger flexors, abductors and opponent muscles of the thumb and the terminal phalanx flexor muscle of the thumb are supplied by the median nerve. In addition, autonomic fibers are contained in the median nerve.

Clinical Presentation of CTS

CTS often presents in early stages with intermittent paresthesias, hyperesthesia, or hypoesthesia in the sensory distribution of the median nerve in the hand. Often, symptoms are first noted in the dominant hand and may be bilateral. Occasionally, complaints are restricted to one or two fingers, usually the middle finger or index and middle fingers. Complaints of pain and numbness may occur later, with up to 15% of affected individuals experiencing pain radiating to the upper arm or shoulder. Symptoms characteristically occur at night and may wake the individual. Many seek relieve by shaking or massaging the hand or by running hot or cold water over the hand. As symptoms progresses, numbness, progressive pain, weakness and atrophy may be experienced. Automatic nerve dysfunction may result in a loss of sweating in areas of the hand innervated by the median nerve. This lack of hand moisture results in a loss of friction when holding objects.

Preventive Measures

Silverstein, Fine and Armstrong outline a strategy of prevention for CTS based on control of known risk factors. The following is adapted from their work:

1. Control of repetition through the use of mechanical aids or automation, job rotation, an increase in work allowances (allowing reasonable rates of work: man-placed instead of machine-placed) or a decrease in production standards, analysis of jobs to eliminate wasted motions, a decrease in overtime, or piecework incentives.
2. Control of force by decreasing the size or weight of objects held, providing tool balances with the center of gravity of the tool aligned with the center of the grasping hand, selecting tools with sufficient hand tool contact area to spread stress evenly over muscles and joints, redesigning tools to use power rather than pinch grip, adding torque bars or dual handles to tools, providing touch-sensitive controls, controlling slipperiness and positioning loads in close and comfortable locations to reduce biomechanical stresses.
3. Control of awkward positions by having adjustable workstations that fit the job to the person, altering the location or orientation of the workstation or work method to allow activity to occur within the normal range of arm movement (decreasing reach, flexion and extension), and redesigning or choosing tools to maintain the wrist in a natural position.
4. Controlling vibration by decreasing the use of impact wrenches and piercing hammers, using dampers and vibration isolators, providing tool balancers, maintaining tool to decreasing cutting resistance and force, purchasing tools with vibration controls, providing adequate rest breaks, controlling the time workers use vibratory tools, and controlling cold exposure.
5. Controlling mechanical stresses by rounding or flaring sharp edges, cushioning tool handles, improving tool purchases and selection, increasing handle length to spread the force over a greater area, providing palm pads, and controlling about the avoidance of using the palm as a hammer.
6. Controlling cold and gloves use problems by providing a variety of gloves sizes and styles which fit well, covering only the part of the hand that is necessary, eliminating gloves whenever possible, controlling ambient temperature, allowing warm-up breaks when working in cold, performing stretching prior to working in the cold, and eliminating the problem of tools exhausting cold air against the hands.

Tendonitis/Tenosynovitis

This is an inflammation of the tendon or the tendon sheath causing inflammation and pain. When inflammation precludes free movement of the finger tendon, the result is stenosing tenosynovitis, or trigger finger. De Quervain's disease results from stenosing tenosynovitis of the abductor pollicis longus and extensor pollicis brevis. Movement which may precipitate these effects include flexion of finger tendons which a flexed wrist (finger flexor tendons); ulnar deviation with outward rotation as in VDT users (finger extensor tendons); or repeated radial or ulnar deviations at the wrist, particularly in combination with force of the thumb (De Quervain's disease). The chronic use of a screwdriver or plier may result in De Quervain's disease.

Epicondylitis

Athletic movements and work tasks may be associated with medial (golfer's elbow) or lateral (tennis elbow) epicondylitis. Contributing activities include wrist/finger extension with elbow extension, abrupt elbow extension or forearm supination as in lifting and pushing up (lateral epicondylitis), or wrist/finger flexion with forearm pronation (medial epicondylitis).

Bicipital/Rotator Cuff Tendinitis

This disorder may be associated with work requiring abduction with or without rotation, as well as constant or repetitive forward elevation of the arm at the shoulder.

Ganglionic Cyst

These may arise after acute trauma or in a degenerative or diseased joint or tendon.

Pronator Syndrome

Proximal forearm pain with pronation of a tightly clenched fist against resistant may be associated with median nerve sensory loss when the median nerve is compressed under the pronator muscle. Repetitious, forceful pronation and finger flexion may cause this syndrome in writers, assembly line workers, or garment workers.

Cubital Tunnel Syndrome

Compare to CTS, ulnar neuropathies at the elbow or forearm may cause more motor and sensory deficit and fewer complaints of pain. This syndrome may be due to entrapment through the cubital tunnel or direct trauma to the nerve at the ulnar groove. Individuals with bilateral symptoms often have shallow ulnar groove. Patient may experience pain, paresthesia, or numbness in the small or ring fingers; difficulty picking up small objects between the thumb and index finger; weak wrist flexion; and atrophy of the hypothenar or interosseous muscles. Tasks associated with repetitive elbow flexion (e.g. hammering and lifting) or repeated trauma or pressure to the ulnar groove (e.g. leaning elbows on a desk or workbench) are possible causal factors.

Ulnar Neuropathy at Guyon's Canal

Motor and sensory symptoms may occur in hand from injury to the palmar branch of the ulnar nerve at the hand/wrist. Using the hand as a hammer or putting pressure on the hypothenar eminence (as in using pneumatic drills) can result in this injury. When the deep motor branch is affected, weakness of the interossei and the third and fourth lumbricales occurs without any sensory findings. This is seen most often in electronics assembly workers, jewelers, and machinists.

Superior or Posterior Interosseous Nerve Syndrome

Single or repeated forceful pronation, supination, radial deviation, or abrupt elbow extension can result in radial nerve compression and injury in the supinator muscle. Affected individuals have weak hand grip and weak wrist/finger extension without sensory symptoms. Musicians, pitchers who throw screwballs, and construction workers who hammer with a straight arm or lift with extended arms are at risk.

Thoracic Outlet Syndrome

Thoracic outlet syndrome may result from either impingement of the blood supply or the nerves to the arm as they pass from the neck to the shoulder. Compression may occur in the scalene muscle, from cervical ribs, fibrous bands, or transverse C7 vertebral process. Symptoms vary with vascular or neurological compression but may include lateral arm pain, paresthesia of the ring and small fingers, hand swelling or weakness. Various activities and postures have been associated with this disorder, including pulling the shoulder back and down, as in military personnel standing at attention, carrying heavy loads in the hand, as in painters, welders, or the persons carrying suitcases and working overhead with repetitive abduction and adduction of the shoulder and arm as in automotive or aircraft repair workers.

Principles of Workstation and Equipment Design that may Reduce the Risk of STI

1. Making workstation easily adjustable and big enough to allow the range of movements required for the job.
2. Reducing static loading of muscles by providing fixtures or jigs to reduce awkward postures and holding the objects by workers.
3. Minimizing force requirements by designing the workstation to provide maximum mechanical advantage to the worker.
4. Reducing contact factors by rounding or padding edges or relocating equipment.
5. Providing seating that gives arm, foot, and back support. Foot rails and antifatigue mats alleviate back stress for standing workers.
6. Selecting tools that minimize risk factors, especially high-contact factors, static loading, awkward hand and finger positions, repetitive finger action, vibration and excessive grip strength requirements.

The use of a video display terminal may involve repetitive upper extremity motions in awkward postures, particularly, if the height and the placement of the chair, desk, computer screen, or keyboard are inappropriate to the worker's size. Static loading of muscles in the upper extremities, neck, shoulders, head and back can also occur. Visual fatigue can result from constant focusing on the computer screen, especially if there is glare from the lighting or bright surfaces in the room. Furthermore, working in a situation in which workers' activities and productivity can be monitored through their computer may exacerbate the physical stresses of the work environment. Concern about the potential health effects of electromagnetic radiation emitted by the terminal, which have not been fully clarify, may induce more stress.

Preventive Measures of Work-related Musculoskeletal Disorders

1. Advice and training, to ensure a higher risk awareness and better working practices.
2. An induction period, to allow new employees to start work at a slower pace than the established workforce.
3. Job rotation or job enlargement to provide respite from work that requires repetitive monotonous use of the same muscles and tendons.
4. Rest breaks. These are often advocated as an alternative to job rotation.
5. A rehabilitation program, to ease affected workers back into productive work.
6. Redeployment.
7. Task optimization. Better design of tools and equipment, and a better work layout make the task easier to perform.

Ergonomics Principles in Material Handling

On the job, ergonomic design of material, container and workstation can help to avoid over-extension and injuries, as should instructions and training on low to 'lift properly'. For some jobs, selection of persons who are physically capable of strenuous material handling may be considered. Material handling is among the most frequent and the most severe causes of injury all over the world. The direct and indirect cost are enormous, and the human suffering associated with, e.g. low back injuries, immeasurable. The following review shows implications for 'ergonomic intervention' to prevent overextensions of material handler, e.g. many lifting instruments including the admonition 'keep the back straight'.

LOW BACK PAIN OF INDUSTRIAL WORKERS

In recent year the requirement for heavy manual labor has decreased dramatically and there is increasing regulation in industries to protect workers. Despite these, there has been a dramatic increase in disability associated with low back pain. This is one of the commonest health hazards in industry. Types of low back pain are:

1. *Mechanical back pain*: About 90% of it accounts to this category. It is due to the overused, traumatized or deformed anatomical structures of the back.
2. *Non-mechanical back pain*: It accounts about 10% of the total back pain cases. It is due to systemic illness.

Occupational (Mechanical) Low Back Pain

Pain in the low back is a major source of incapacitation among working people. Because low back pain is such a complex medical problem, it is frequently difficult to relate the low back problem to injury. Persisting low back pain is recognized as chronic when symptoms persist longer than 3 months. In the majority of the cases, the back pain is called non-specific because the cause of the pain cannot be located with current diagnostic methods. Because the pain is mostly felt in the lower part of the back, the back pain is also termed 'low back pain'. Back pain is limiting in activities where posture must be maintained for a long-time (such as standing or sitting) and carrying out specific movement (such as lifting, bending or walking). In turn, limitation of these activities leads to work disability and the restriction of participation in other important activities. A NIOSH review of epidemiological research on low back pain and occupational risk factors with 42 studies up to 1997 concluded that there was strong evidence for an association between lifting and forceful movement and back disorders. Pre-existing depression or psychological problems, workplace dissatisfaction, contentious compensation claims, and even other type of chronic pain may be present.

Back disorders can develop gradually as a result of microtrauma brought about by repetitive activity over time or can be the product of a single traumatic event. Because of the slow and progressive onset of this internal injury, the condition is often ignored until the symptoms become acute, often resulting in disabling injury. Acute back injury can be the immediate result of improper lifting techniques and/or lifting loads that are too heavy for the back to support. While the acute injury may seem to be caused by a single well-defined incident, the real cause is often a combined interaction of the observed stressors coupled with years of weakening of the musculoskeletal support mechanism by repetitive microtrauma. Injuries can arise in muscle, ligament, and discs, either singly or in combination.

Although back injuries account for no work-related deaths, they do account for a significant amount of human suffering, loss of productivity, and economic burden on compensation systems. Back disorders are one of the leading causes of disability for people in their working years and afflict over 600000 employees each year with a cost of about $50 annually in 1991 according to NIOSH. The frequency and economic impact of back injuries and disorders on the workforce are expected to increase over the next several decades as the average age of the workforce increases and medical cost go up.

Factors Associated with Back Disorders

Back disorders result from exceeding the capability of the muscles, tendons, discs, or the cumulative effect of several contributors:

1. Reaching while lifting.
2. Poor posture—how one sits or stands.
3. Stressful living and working activities—staying in one position for too long.
4. Bad body mechanics—how one lifts, pushes, pulls, or carries objects.
5. Poor physical condition—losing the strength and endurance to perform physical tasks without strain.
6. Poor design of job or workstation.
7. Repetitive lifting of awkward items, equipment, or (in healthcare facilities) patients.
8. Twisting while lifting.
9. Bending while lifting.
10. Maintaining bent posture.
11. Heavy lifting.
12. Fatigue.
13. Poor footing such as slippery floors, or constrained posture.
14. Lifting with forceful movement.
15. Vibration, such as with lift truck driver, delivery drivers, etc.

Signs and Symptoms

Signs and symptoms include pain when attempting to assume normal posture, decreased mobility, and pain when standing or rising from a seated position.

Contributing Factors of Back Injuries

These factors usually account for very few work-related back injuries:

1. Congenital defects of the spine.
2. Increase in static standing or sitting tasks.
3. An aging workforce.
4. Decreases in physical conditioning and exercise.
5. Job dissatisfaction.

Risks of Low Back Pain due to Manual Material Handling

Major need in occupational medicine is to identify risk factors for the development of work-related low back pain associated with materials handling. This will allow us to tailor job tasks to the physical capacity of industrial workers and design industrial production methods that do not exceed the physical abilities of the majority of the workforce. If we adopt the strategy, future incidence of work-related back pain may begin to decline. We have to consider the following factors:

1. *Medical history*: One of the most important parts of pre-placement medical history deals with previous musculoskeletal problem. A prior history of low-back pain is a significant predictive risk factor for subsequent work-related low-back pain. Up to 80% of the population will experience an episode of low-back pain during their lifting. Recurrent episodes appear to be part of the natural history of the disease in many individuals.
2. *Physical examination*: The physical examination can show signs of dysfunction indicative of inability to perform certain job tasks and findings associated with a risk of future problems.
3. *Radiographic examination*: Pre-placement X-ray of the lumbar spines are done to screen workers for the development of low-back pain and injury in the workplace.
4. *Strength testing*: Strength testing has been widely used in industry over the past few decades to screen job applicants for ability to perform lifting tasks and to predict the risk of future low-back pain. The goal of this test has been to assure that only people with sufficient strength to perform a job safely be assigned to that job. Methods tested include isometric, isokinetic, isoinertial, psychophysical, and dynamic work-capacity evaluations.
5. *Fitness and training*: There is some evidence that individuals with a good state of general fitness have less risk of chronic low-back pain than others and that recovery after a pain episode is faster in these subjects.
6. *Lifting technique*: Several lifting techniques have been recommended in the past. The most common recommendation is to lift with the back straight and knees bend while using the leg muscles. Squat lifting has been observed to produce smaller compressive forces on the lumbar spine, probably because it moves the load closer to the spinal axis.
7. *Job factors*: It must be recognized that causation of low-back pain is very difficult to establish because of the episodic nature of the symptoms. In fact, referring low-back pain as an 'injury' is not doing justice to the complexity of the problem. Snook et al estimated that 70% of the low-back injuries are associated with lifting act. Chaffin and Park found that persons performing >150 lifts per day had an increased risk of low-back pain. Lifting associated with bending and twisting is felt to be the most frequent cause of low-back pain. A NIOSH panel of investigators has identified several task factors as risks in lifting. These include load weight, horizontal distance from the spinal axis, vertical distance from the floor, distance displaced, frequency and duration of lifting, asymmetry of the lift, and the quality of the coupling between the hand and the load. Pushing and pulling are associated with 9–18% of the back strains and sprains. Prolong sitting has been identified as a risk of low-back pain, as has vibration transmitted from tools, motor vehicles, and resonating platform or floor.

Control of Back injuries

1. Alter the task to eliminate the hazardous motion and/or change the position of the object in relation to the employee's body, such as adjusting the height of the pallet or shelf.
2. Material handling tasks should be designed to minimize the weight, range of motion, and frequency of activity.
3. Work methods and stations should be designed to minimize the distance between the person and the object being handled.

4. Platforms and conveyors should be built at about waist height to minimize awkward postures. Conveyors or carts should be used for horizontal motion whenever possible. Reduce the size or weight of the object(s) lifted.
5. High-strength push-pull requirements are undesirable, but pulling is better than pushing. Material handling equipment should be easy to move, with handles that can be easily grasped in an upright posture.
6. Workbench or workstation configurations can force people to bend over. Corrections should emphasize adjustments necessary for the employee to remain in a relaxed upright stance or fully supported seated posture. Bending the upper body and spine to reach into a bin or container is highly undesirable. The bins should be elevated, tilted or equipped with collapsible sides to improve access.
7. Repetitive or sustained twisting, stretching, or leaning to one side are undesirable. Corrections could include repositioning bins and moving employees closer to parts and conveyors.
8. Store heavy objects at waist level.
9. Provide lift-assist devices, and lift tables.
10. Work training and education:
    a. Training should include general principles of ergonomics, recognition of hazards and injuries, procedures for reporting hazardous conditions, and methods and procedures for early reporting of injuries. Additionally, job specific training should be given on safe work practices, hazards, and controls.
    b. Strength and fitness training.
11. Rotating of employees, providing a short break every hour, or using a two person lift may be helpful.
12. Rotation is not simply a different job, but must be a job that utilizes a completely different muscle group from the ones that have been over-exerted.
13. Standing for extended periods places excessive stress on the back and legs. Solutions include a footrest or rail, resilient floor mats, height-adjustable chairs or stools, and opportunities for the employee to change position.
14. Where employees are seated the chairs or stools must be properly chosen.
15. Proper adjustable lumbar support may be provided.
16. Static seated posture with bending or reaching should be avoided.

Occupational Health Survey

Purpose

Assist in identifying new or early cases of back injury and disorders in the workforce. Useful in smaller facilities where data gathered from records review may be limited or in facilities where reporting disincentives limit the number of reported cases. The major reason for this is to collect data on the number of workers that may be experiencing some form of back injury or disorder. This is also a good method for identifying departments or jobs where potential back problems exist.

Mass Medical Screening

Mass medical screening could be useful but must be performed by trained medical staff.

Job Analysis and Observation

Each job in which workers have a greater incidence of back disorders might be subject to a job analysis after an appropriate records review and workers survey.

Work-Method Analysis

1. Observe employees at work: Notice what employees are doing to make themselves more comfortable in the workplace. Watch for repeated motions and the position of the arms, wrist and trunk (e.g. overstretching or unusual posture).
2. Record the movements used to perform the task. Used a video camera for subsequent slow-motion analysis.
3. An ergonomic checklist can be helpful on inspections to record information which is not readily identifiable from the videotape; and (40 workstation and tool evaluation may be necessary.

Prevention of Low Back Pain

Pre-employment strength testing and ergonomic job design together were seen as the most promising intervention methods. It appears possible to control back pain by reducing the probability of the initial episode, reducing the length of the disability, and reducing the chance of recurrence. Realization of these goals was deemed possible with a combination of job design, job placement and education/training. The important preventive measures for low-back pain:

1. *Exposure limits*: If spinal loading at work is a main risk factor for back pain, then it makes sense to try to reduce spinal load by setting maximum permissible limits. According to the American National Institute of Occupational Safety and Health (NIOSH), the maximum recommended weight limit is 23 kg (51 pounds).
2. *Workplace improvements, participatory ergonomics*: Ergonomic improvements may improve comfort and efficiency.
3. *Pre-employment examination*: It is possible to reduce health problems of low back pain through pre-employment selection.
4. *Work education and training*: Workers should be trained to perform their work appropriately and safely. Educational programs try to increase knowledge on the causes of back pain, often in combination with exercise to improve function or physical fitness.
5. *Exercise*: The following three mechanisms are held responsible for the preventive effect of exercise:
   a. Strengthening of back muscles and increasing trunk flexibility.
   b. Increasing the blood supply to the spine muscles, joints, and intervertebral discs.
   3. Improving mood and thereby altering the perception of pain.

KEYBOARDS AND MUSCULOSKELETAL DISORDERS

Problems in the continuous use of keyboards have been described by the workers/users. Forguson describes 'telegraphists cramps and myalgia': Duncan, Ferguson and Kroemer further expand on this subject with experimentally obtained results from individuals working with keyboards. Duncan and Ferguson obtained medical results from faulty body positions versus keyboard operations and concluded that body positions of extended periods of shoulder abduction (elbow away from body), ulnar deviation of the wrist (palm down, hand turned outward) and wrist extension (palm down, back of hand turned upward) were important predictors of keyboard operators' medical symptoms.

Repetition is a factor in cumulative trauma disorders. The modern information procession system provides many functions that eliminate manual interruptions previously needed in keyboarding work, thus enhancing the rate and quantity of key strokes and uninterrupted duration at keyboarding work.

While the force needed to activate keys is not likely to stress the musculoskeletal systems of the hand and wrist, high repetition rates and long-duration keying performed at awkward positions may be sufficient to cause MSDs in susceptible individuals.

A review of the ergonomic of keyboard design leads to suggested keyboard designs and use that could change keying positions and reduce symptoms as follows:

1. To correct shoulder abduction, the keyboard should be positioned near the front edge of the table and be movable so that it can be turned in a horizontal plane.
2. To correct ulnar deviation, having the keyboard in a movable horizontal plane is of importance.
3. To correct pronation and extension of the wrist, the keyboard should have a tilt.
4. Means for periodic support or rest of the arms, wrist, and hands should be provided.
5. All surfaces which contact arms, wrist, and hands should be free of hard or cutting edges.
6. Task should be varied in terms of motion patterns or rest breaks or relief activities provided.
7. Operators need to be trained in the hand/wrist postures that minimize the probability of musculoskeletal disorders.

VISUAL DISPLAY TERMINALS (VDTS) AND VISION

Prolonged, intensive use of VDTs can cause eyestrain, irritation, blurred vision, and headache. Many individuals have a need for their vision to be corrected. The viewing distance involved in VDT use may require corrective eyeglasses different from those use for everyday activities. For example, wearers of bifocals who use the reading portion of their lenses to view the display may force their neck into an awkward position which strains their neck and shoulder muscles.

Concentration on the VDT screen tends to reduce blinking, which can dry eyes, particularly for those who wear contact lens. Dry eye can feel gritty, tired, and irritated. Raising the viewing position of the screen can result in more eye surface exposure, resulting in another cause for eye dryness and reduce blink rate. Users should blink more frequently and take occasional eye rests (a momentary change is all that is required).

The screen is itself a reflective surface and so screen glare caused by reflected light from windows, incorrectly positioned lighting, and shiny work surfaces are a common cause of eyestrain. The screen should be positioned relative to windows, overhead lights, and other glare sources to minimize these reflections. Indirect lighting will help to so minimize those reflections and appropriate individual task lights can be used for illuminating working copy. Poorly formed images (characters, shapes) on the screen will also cause eyestrain. The American National Standard Institute (ANSI) and International Standard Organization (ISO) have issued standards for the design of VDTs to provide satisfactory front-screen characteristics and to minimize visual discomfort.

SEDENTARY WORK AND CHAIR DESIGN

Since such work is done sitting down, and much of it for extended periods, implications for sedentary work should be considered. Mankind is not fully adapted to being an erect, two-footed animal and is even more maladapted to evolved sitting arrangements. Sitting can put more strain on the lower spine than standing the intervertebral disc pressure while seated and keyboarding can be twice that of standing at ease.

A well-designed chair for the operator is one of the most important parts of a workstation. It can favorably affect posture, circulation, the amount of effort required to maintain a position, and the amount of pressure on the spine.

The following recommendations should be followed:

1. The seat should adapt to the user, not *vice versa*.
2. Chairs should be stable and fully and easily adjustable from the seated position.
3. Seat pans and backrests should be upholstered and covered in a material which absorbs perspiration. They should be firm, with a compression of about 20 mm.
4. Seat pan height should be adjustable and should transfer the user's weight through the buttocks, not the thighs.
5. Backrests should adjust up and down and backward and forward for good lumbar support.
6. Where mobility is required, wheels or casters should be fitted to the chair (hard casters for soft floors and soft casters for hard floors). There are exceptions to this, e.g. where a slippery floor makes it difficult to keep the chair in the desired position. Where wheels or casters are fitted, seats should preferably have five legs. This offers improved stability and reduces the risk of tipping over.
7. Seating should provide sufficient clearance for the flesh of the thigh in order to prevent reduction of blood circulation. The front of the seat should be of a 'waterfall' design.
8. For tasks requiring frequent lateral movements, seats should swivel.

The work in very different applications, of Mandal, Grandjean, et al. and Andersson, et al. shows that the classical orthogonal (all joints at right angles) seated position is not the optimum. They add support to these recommendations, the final recommendation being the adjustable, reclining back chair.

Sitting is an act. A pattern of behavior that varies in time and space depending on: task, duration, discretion, physical configuration of the chair; relation of the chair to work surfaces; physical and psychological state of the user; demographics of the user. Research into the analysis and evaluation of occupational seating is now underway. The followings are the actions to improve the effectiveness of, and minimize the probability of musculoskeletal disorders of the sedentary worker:

1. Tune the musculoskeletal system (exercise)
2. Use proper posture:
   a. Adjust chair and workstation
   b. Use backrest
   c. Feet flat on floor (may be footrest)
   d. Change posture
   e. Always support/assist the back
   f. Articulated back support (angle between spine and seat about 110°)

g. Share load with feet and legs
h. Job design for postural pauses
i. Health education.

3. Ergonomic chair and workstation:
   a. Easily adjusted from seated position
   b. Seat pan height adjustable
   c. Seat pan depth about two-thirds of thigh length
   d. Seat pan and backrest—compression and material to specifications
   e. Backrest—lumbar support height and pressure adjustable
   f. Seat pan angle adjustable with compensated backrest
   g. Working surface/space at appropriate height/position.

POSTURE AND WORKSTATION DESIGN

Postural fixity can occur because the fixed position of the screen results in a fixed head position and trunk immobility or the automated nature of the system results in limited hand and arm movements and limited need for postural changes.

Awkward postures can occur because an improper match between work-surface height and user position can cause increased musculoskeletal stresses of forearm and upper arm; inadequate work surfaces can result in musculoskeletal stresses of neck and shoulders and unnecessary arm and hand movements; improper height of screen and inadequate vision correction can cause undue musculoskeletal stresses of neck and shoulder; improper positioning and use of the keyboard can result in awkward ulnar and radial deviations and extension and flexion of the wrists.

Ancillary equipment such as a footrest to assist in accommodating chair, table height, and human adjustment, a wrist/arm rest, and individual task lighting for working document illumination should be considered.

The design of workstation, its environment and its ancillary equipment, is important to alleviating musculoskeletal discomforts and disorders.

Chapter

4

Personal Protective Equipment

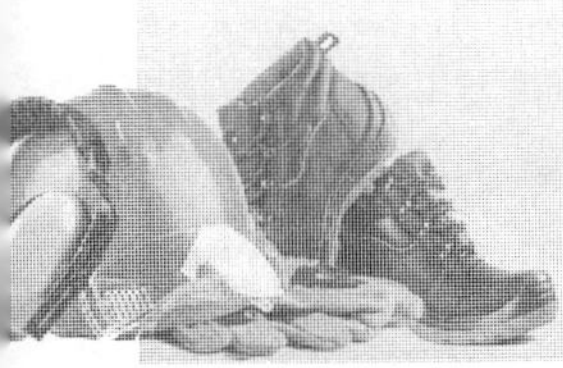

Personal protective equipment is a device which is designed to interpose effective barrier between a person and harmful objects, substances or deviations recommended for use in industrial operation/process, mines, construction work, etc. associated with hazardous jobs. It must be born in mind that the PPE does not eliminate a hazard but minimizes it. It also provides second line of protection.

Legal Requirement

In the Factories Act, 1948 there are specific provisions for providing the personal protect equipment to the workers who are exposed to unsafe and unhealthy environment. The provisions of law relating to use of personal protective equipment in different operations and processes are framed in such a spirit that the workers working on the operations and in processes are protected against possible hazards. It is also the intention of the law that the personal protective equipment shall be of such type and made of such materials that withstand to such specific hazards for which it is being used.

Need for Personal Protective Equipment

In industry it may be possible to substitute a dangerous substance with a safer substance isolate the process, to have automatic and mechanical handling of the substance or to controlled ventilation of the process or to plan and arrange operation that personal protective equipment is not necessary, but sometimes it may not be possible to introduce such measures or there might be a breakdown in the plant or in the control measure. Under such circumstances it will become necessary to use personal protective equipment. It must be borne in mind the personal protective equipment does not eliminate a hazard. These devices designed to interpose an effective barrier between a person and harmful objects, substances, or deviations.

Requirements of suitable personal protective equipment can be listed as under:

- Nature of the hazard.
- Severity of the hazard.
- Type of contaminant.
- Concentration of the contaminants.
- Duration of work.
- Location of the contaminated area with respect to a source of respirable air.
- Expected activity of the wearer.

– Operating characteristic and limitations of the equipment.
– Reliability of the equipment.
– Acceptance of the wearer.
– Cost of equipment.

Role of PPE

a. Acts as barrier between man and hazardous objects/exposure.
b. Provides cushioning effect against impact loading.
c. Supplies fresh/pure air in contaminated atmosphere.
d. Protect important/vital body parts.
e. Reduces severity of injury/health hazard.
f. Acts as a last resort and not a substitute for engineering control.

TYPES OF PERSONAL PROTECTIVE EQUIPMENT

Personal protective equipment may be divided into two broad groups:

1. Non-respiratory Personal Protective Equipment

Personal protective equipment for various parts of the body can be divided into six broad groups:

a. Head Protection

Head protectors may be hard hats and caps made of aluminum, PVC fiber glass, laminated plastic or valcunized fiber. They may be fitted with brackets for fixing welding masks protective face screen, or a lamp. The hats and caps are provided with replaceable hardness which provides sufficient clearance between the top of the head and shell.

Equipment: Hats, caps and helmets

Material	*Hazard*
Asbestos	Sparks, hot materials, heat
Plastic rubber	Hot liquids, moisture, acids, alkalis, electric shocks and dermatitis
Cotton wool	Sparks and heat, dermatitis and machinery
Metal	Falling objects, flying particles, cuts and abrasions
Plastic	Sparks, falling objects, flying particles, electrical shock, cuts and abrasions

Safe caps and hoods are also used for protection against heat, spark, and other dangerous materials and are made of appropriate materials. Sometimes hoods are made with rigid frame which is held away from the head.

b. Eye and Face Protection

There are no reliable statistics but the eye injuries account for about 5% of all industrial injuries and 50% of the cases seen in an eye hospital. The eye injuries are caused due to:

a. Flying objects	80%
b. Tools or parts of machinery	8%
c. Splashes of liquid	7%
d. Explosive	2.5%
e. Falls	2%
f. Infection	0.5%

Numerous eye injuries are caused by dusts, flying particles, splashes and harmful radiations. It is difficult to precisely cover the various processes in which the workers may be required to wear goggles. The hazards encountered may be:

1. *Relatively large flying objects*: Chipping, felting, riveting, sledging, caulking, etc.
2. *Dust and small flying objects*: Scaling, grinding, stone dressing, wood-working.
3. *Splashing of metals*: Pouring of lead joints, casting of metals, galvanizing and dirpping in molten metals.
4. *Splashing of liquids gases and fumes:* Handling of acids and other chemicals.
5. *Reflected light glare and radiant energy*: Foundry work, glass furnaces, gas welding and cutting arc welding.

Eye Protectors

1. Safety spectacles
2. Mono-goggles
3. Impact goggles
4. Chemical goggles
5. Gas tight goggles
6. Face shields
7. Welding helmets
8. Welding goggles
9. Foundry goggles.

c. Hand and Arm Protector

Protection of hands and arm becomes necessary when workers have to handle materials having sharp and sharp edges or when hot and molten metals, chemicals and corrosive substances have to be handled. The protective equipment may be gauntlet gloves, wrist gloves, mittens, hand pads and thumb and finger guards and sleeves. It is important not only that the various parts of arm and hand are adequately covered, but that they should be covered by a material suitable for withstanding the specific hazard involved:

Equipment: Sleeves, wristlets

Material	*Hazard*
Asbestos	Sparks, hot materials and heat
Chrome leathers	Sparks, hot materials, hot liquids, flying particles, cuts and abrasions.
Flame proofed duck	Sparks, hot materials, heat flying particles, and machinery.
Plastic	Hot liquids, moisture, acids and alkalis, electric shock and dermatitis
Rubber	Hot liquids, moisture, acids and alkalis, and dermatitis
Chemical materials	Acids and alkalis
Reflective fabric	Hot liquids

Equipment: Gloves, mittens, hand pads and finger guards:

Material	*Hazard*
Asbestos	Sparks, hot materials and heat
Chrome leather	Sparks, hot materials, hot liquids, flying particles, cuts and abrasions
Rubber	Hot liquids, moisture, acids and alkalis, electric shock and dermatitis
Plastic	Hot liquids, moisture, acids and alkalis and dermatitis
Metal mesh	Cuts and abrasions
Cotton	Cuts and abrasions

d. Foot and Leg Protection

Adequate protection may have to be provided to the workers employed in certain jobs. Risk of injury may be in handling of heavy materials, caustic and corrosive liquids, wet conditions, molten metals, etc. Common foot and leg protective equipment are safety shoes and boots, leggings, foot-guards and leg guards.

Equipment: Knee pads, leggings

Material	*Hazard*
Asbestos	Sparks, hot materials and heat
Chrome leather	Sparks, hot materials, hot liquids, flying particles, cuts and abrasions.
Flame proofed duck	Sparks, hot materials, heat flying particles, and machinery.
Plastic	Hot liquids, moisture, acids and alkalis and dermatitis
Rubber	Hot liquids, moisture, acids and alkalis, electric shock and dermatitis.
Fibre metal	Sparks, flying objects, flying particles, cuts, abrasions and machinery
Chemical resistant	Acids and alkalis
Reflective fabric	Hot liquids

Equipment: Shoes and boots

Material	*Hazard*
Steel toe caps	Falling objects
Non-skid shoes	Moisture
Wooden soles	Hot materials, heat, hot liquids, moisture, acids and alkalis, slips and falls, and cuts and abrasions
Chrome leather	Sparks, hot materials, heat and hot liquids.
Rubber	Hot liquids, moisture, acids and alkalis, electric-shock and dermatitis
Conductive rubber	Explosive

e. Body Protection

Sometimes it becomes necessary to provide special protective equipment for the body in the form of aprons, over-all, jackets and complete head to toe protective suits. Nature of potential hazard, degree of the hazard involved and nature of activities of the user concerned are important considerations in the selection of safety clothing. Although complete coverage of the body and legs is not needed in many cases and unnecessary safety clothing may hamper the efficiency of the user, no compromise should be made with strict safety requirements. If a user needs complete coverage, he should have it.

Equipment: Coats, aprons and overall jacket, complete head to toe protective suit, waist:

Material	*Hazard*
Asbestos	Sparks, hot materials and heat
Chrome leather	Sparks, hot materials, hot liquids, flying particles, cuts and abrasions.
Plastic	Hot liquids, moisture, acids and alkalis, electric shock, dermatitis and machinery
Rubber	Hot liquids, moisture, acids and alkalis, electric shock, dermatitis, machinery
Canvas	Flying particles, cuts and abrasions and machinery
Chemical resistant fabric	Acids and alkalis
Reflective fabric	Hot liquids

f. Ear Protection

There are situations in which noise reduction or control techniques are impractical or insufficient. In this situations, personal hearing protection must be used. An effective PPE serves as a barrier between the noise and the inner ear where noise-induced damage to hearing may occur. Ear protector devices usually take the form of ear muffs which are worn over the external ear and provide an acoustic seal against the head, or ear plugs which provide an acoustical seal at the entrance to the external ear canal. Therefore, ear protection provides a system of attenuation of the incoming sound and thus minimizes the sound arriving at the tympanic membrane. If the ear protectors are not fitted properly or are of poor quality, then the sound energy may reach the inner ear of persons wearing protectors by four different pathways and they are (Fig. 4.1):

1. By passing through bone and tissue around the protectors.
2. By causing vibration of the protector which in turn generates sound into the external ear.
3. By passing through leaks in the protector.
4. By passing through leaks around the protector.

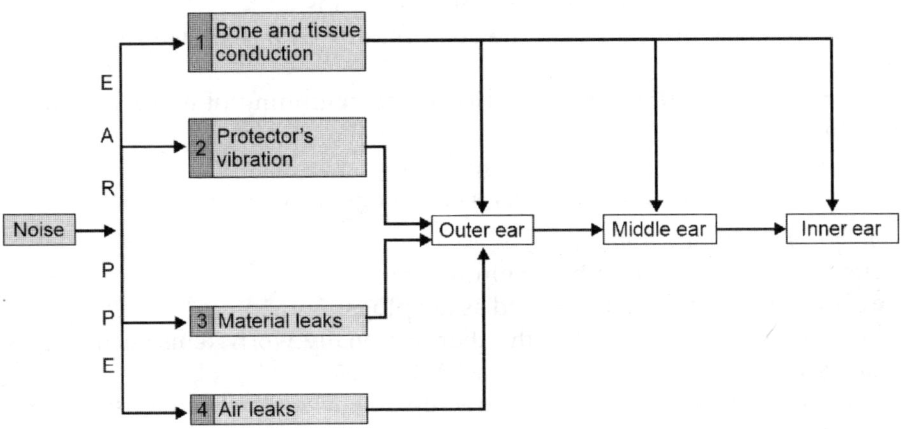

Fig. 4.1: Pathway to bypass ear protectors

The following rules should be observed to minimize losses due to acoustic leaks:

1. Ear protector should be made of imperforated materials.
2. The protector should be designed to conform readily to the head or ear canal configuration so that an efficient acoustic seal can be worn with reasonable comfort.
3. The protector should have a support means or a seal compliance that will minimize protector vibration.
4. Muff-type protector should not be worn over long hair, thick and/or poorly fitted eye-glass temples, or other obstacles.

Various types of ear protectors:

Earmuff: Earmuffs fit over the ears and are sealed to the side of the head by a soft cushion seals filled with soft plastic foam or a viscous fluid. They are usually held in position by means of a headband but may alternatively be attached to a soft helmet. Attenuation may be 'frequency selective', protecting some frequencies more than others, particularly the higher frequencies rather than the speech frequencies. 'Amplitude selective' devices are designed to provide attenuation that increases with sound level. Such a device usually has a small hole which acts as a mechanical filter, allowing low sound pressures to pass but offering more resistance at high pressures. 'Active devices' incorporate electronic circuitry which limits the transmission of sound at high intensity and are of value when workers are exposed to short burst of high intensity sound or impulsive sounds. 'Anti-noise' devices incorporate circuitry which cancels out incident noise especially at low frequency. These devices are still largely experimental. Many of the newer muffs incorporate an in-built communication system.

While the ear muffs usually provide an effective level of attenuation, their value may be limited by any effect which decreases the efficiency of the seal, e.g. spectacle frames, goggles, beards and long-hair, or scarves worm under the muffs. Furthermore, wear and tear may decrease the efficiency of the seal. It should also be emphasized that if protection is removed in noisy areas, even for a short period, the amount of protection will be severely limited, e.g. if a protector with an 'assumed protection' of 20 dB(A) is removed for 30 minutes per day the actual reduction in noise dose received by the wearer will be only 12 dB(A).

Advantages of the use of ear muffs:

1. The protection provided by a good ear muff is generally greater and less variable between wearers than that of good ear plug.
2. A single size of ear muff fits a large percentage of heads.
3. The relatively large muff size can be seen readily at a distance for the purpose of monitoring.
4. Muffs are usually accepted more readily at the beginning of a hearing conservation program than ear plugs.
5. Muffs can be worn even with minor ear infection.
6. Muffs are not misplaced or lost as easily as ear plugs.

Disadvantages of the use of ear muffs:

1. Ear muffs are uncomfortable in hot environment.
2. They are not as easily carried nor stored as ear plugs.
3. Ear muffs are not as compatible with other personally worn items such as glasses and headgear as are ear plugs.
4. The relatively large muff size may not be acceptable when the head must be maneuvered in closed quarters.
5. Ear muffs are more expensive.

Ear plug: Ear plugs are generally thought to be less efficient attenuators of sound than muffs, but have the advantage that they are easy to use. They may be disposable or permanent. Disposable plugs are made of a compressible or conformable material. They are readily available commercially, but have a finite 'life expectancy' after which their effectiveness decreases. Permanent and custom moulded plugs have a longer survival, and are usually comfortable if made by an experienced technician. One of the main disadvantages of plugs is the increased propensity to otitis externa, although this too can occur with muffs. Dual protection with the use of both muffs and ear plugs may be indicated when the noise levels are extremely high (when L_{EPd} exceeds about 115 dBA).

Advantages of the use of ear plugs:

1. Ear plugs are small and carried easily.
2. They can be worn conveniently and efficiently with other personally worn items such as glasses, headgear or hairstyles.
3. Ear plugs are relatively comfortable to wear in hot environment.
4. They are convenient to wear where the head must be maneuvered in closed quarters.
5. The cost of the ear plug is significantly less than muff.

Disadvantages of the use of ear plugs:

1. Ear plugs require more time and effort for fitting than for muffs.
2. The amount of protection provided by a good earplug is generally less than ear muffs.
3. Dirt may be inserted into the ear canal if an ear plug is removed and reinserted with dirty hands.
4. Ear plugs are difficult to see in the ear from a distance for the purpose of monitoring.
5. Ear plugs can be worn only in healthy ear canal.

Hearing Protective Helmets (Noise-excluding Helmets)

An extremely high levels of sound (in tunnelling), the protection offered by muffs and plugs, either alone or in combination, may be insufficient. Sound may still reach the ears through nose, mouth, eye sockets and the skull itself. The attenuation provided by the protector should comply with British Standard BS 510866 (ISO 4869), and the basic design features should comply with BS 6344. The 'assumed protection' of a device will vary with frequency and most will attenuate higher frequency sound better than low frequency sound. The 'assumed protection level' of noise exposure is obtained by subtracting the assumed protection of the device at each octave band frequency from the sound pressure level at each frequency.

Other Types of Hearing Protectors

a. Selective attenuated for high frequency: For musician.
b. Selective attenuated for high intensity: For pistol/rifle shooters.

2. Respiratory Personal Protective Equipment

History of the Development of Respiratory Protection

The concept of using respiratory protective devices to reduce or eliminate hazardous exposures to airborne contaminants first came from Pliny (circa AD 23-79) who discussed the idea of using loose fitting animal bladders in roman mines to protect workers from the inhalation of red oxide of lead. Later in the 1700's, the ancestors of modern atmosphere-supplying devices, such as the self-contained breathing apparatus or hose mask, were developed. Although the devices themselves have become more sophisticated in design and materials, respirators' performance is still based on one of the two basic principles: purifying the air by removing contaminants before they reach the breathing zone of the worker, or providing clean air from an uncontaminated source.

In 1814, a particulate-removing filter encased in a rigid container was developed—the predecessor of modern filters for air-purifying respirators. In 1854, it was recognized that activated charcoal could be used as a filtering medium for vapors. During World War I, with the use of chemical warfare, improvements of the design of respirators was necessary. In 1930, the development of the resin-impregnated dust filter made available efficient, inexpensive filters that have good dust-loading characteristics and low breathing resistance.

A more recent development was the high efficiency particulate filter made with very fine glass fibers. These extremely efficient filters are used for very small airborne particles and produce little breathing resistance. Some features that are currently being incorporated into respirator design include a smaller face-piece, which translates into a better field of vision and a low profile that permits the respirator to fit under other protective gear such as welder's helmet. Over the years there have been continuing major developments in the basic design of respirators. Modern design improvements have created products that are both more comfortable to wear and more protective than earlier.

Introduction

Personal protective equipment (PPE) is a device which is designed to interpose as effective barrier between a person and harmful objects, substances or deviations recommended for use in industrial operation/process, mines, construction work, etc. associated with hazardous jobs. It must be born in mind that the PPE does not eliminate a hazard but minimizes it. Personal protective equipment is divided into two groups—respiratory and non-respiratory.

Atmospheric contaminants range from the relatively harmless substances to toxic dusts fumes, smokes, mists, vapor and gases. Processes which present hazards of exposure to harmful substances should, if possible, be closed or ventilated to eliminate or minimize the hazard. If enclosure, ventilation or other engineering means of control are not possible or become very costly to apply to the degree required to ensure absolute safety, respirator equipment should be provided to the workers exposed to possible hazard. Even though engineering measures of control are applied satisfactorily, a supply of appropriate protective equipment should be readily available for use, as there will be plant breakdowns and repair may have to be carried out in contaminated environments. Respiratory protective equipment should be considered a last resort, or as stand by protection and never a substitute for effective engineering control:

A. Wearing respiratory protective devices to reduce exposure to airborne contaminants is widespread in industry. An estimated 5 million workers wear respirators, either occasionally or routinely. Although it is preferred industrial hygiene practice to use engineering controls to reduce contaminants emissions at their source, there are operations where this type of control is not technologically or economically feasible or is otherwise inappropriate.

B. Since respirators are not as consistently reliable as engineering and work practice controls, and may create additional problem, they are not the preferred method of reducing exposures below the occupational exposure levels. Accordingly, their use as a primary control is restricted to certain circumstances. In those circumstances where engineering and work practice control cannot be used to reduce airborne contaminants below their occupational exposure levels (e.g. certain maintenance and repair operation, emergencies, or during periods when engineering controls are being installed), the use of respirators could be justified to reduce worker exposure. In other cases, where work practices and engineering controls alone cannot reduce exposure levels below the occupational exposure level, the use of respirators would be essential for supplemental protection.

C. There are many variables that the degree of protection afforded by respiratory protection devices, and the misuse of respirators can be hazardous to employee safety and health. Selection of the wrong equipment, one of the most frequent errors made in respiratory protection, can result in the employee using exposure to increased concentrations of the harmful contaminant. This error may result in a broad range of health effects caused by the harmful contaminants, including silicosis, permanent lung damage, and cancer. Respirators that are not maintained and inspected can be less effective at reducing exposure to the harmful contaminants, and can place a greater burden on the respiratory system. Respirator, i.e. not clean can cause dermatitis or skin irritation. Because respirator use may be given the employee a false sense of security and presumed protection, an improper respirator program can actually present a high degree of hazard for the employee.

D. Respirators can only provide adequate protection if they are properly selected for the task; are fitted to the wearer and are consistently donned and worn properly; and are properly maintained so that they continue to provide the protection required for the work situation. These variables can only be controlled if a comprehensive respiratory protection program is developed and implemented in each workplace where respirators are used. When respirator use is augmented by an appropriate respiratory protection program, it can prevent fatalities and illness from both acute and chronic exposures to hazardous substances.

Type of Respirators According to their Fitting

The purpose of a respirator is to prevent the inhalation of harmful airborne substances and/or an oxygen-deficient atmosphere. Functionally, a respirator is designed as an enclosure that covers the nose and mouth or the entire face or head. Respirators are of two general 'fit' types, tight-fitting and loose-fitting.

1. *The tight-fitting respirator*: This is designed to form a seal with the face of the wearer. It is available in three types: quarterly mask, half mask, and full face-piece (Fig. 4.2). The quarter mask covers the nose and mouth, where the lower sealing surface rests between the chin and the mouth. The half mask covers the nose and mouth and fits under the chin. The full face-piece covers the entire face from below the chin to the hairline.

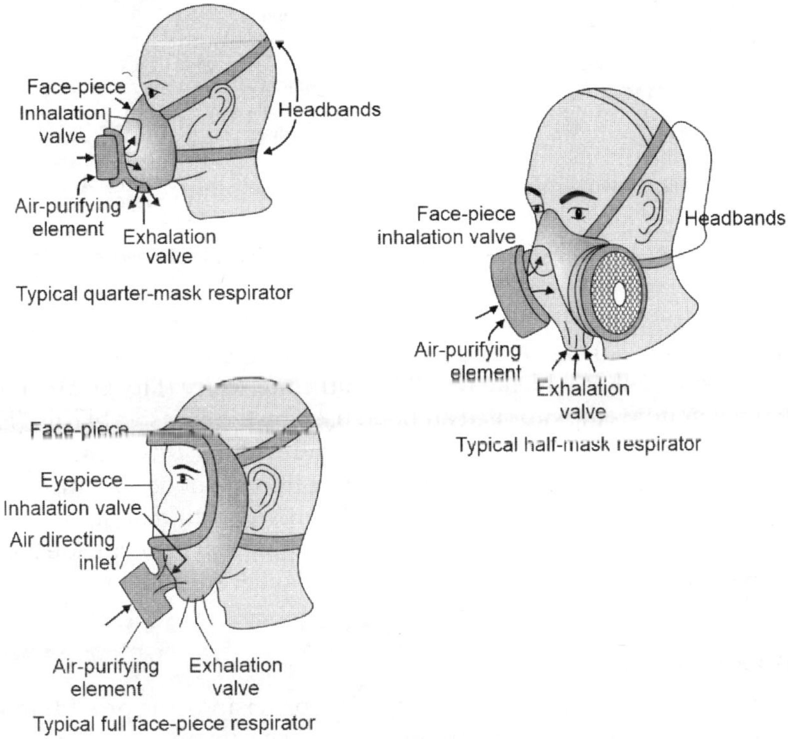

Fig. 4.2: Types of respirators

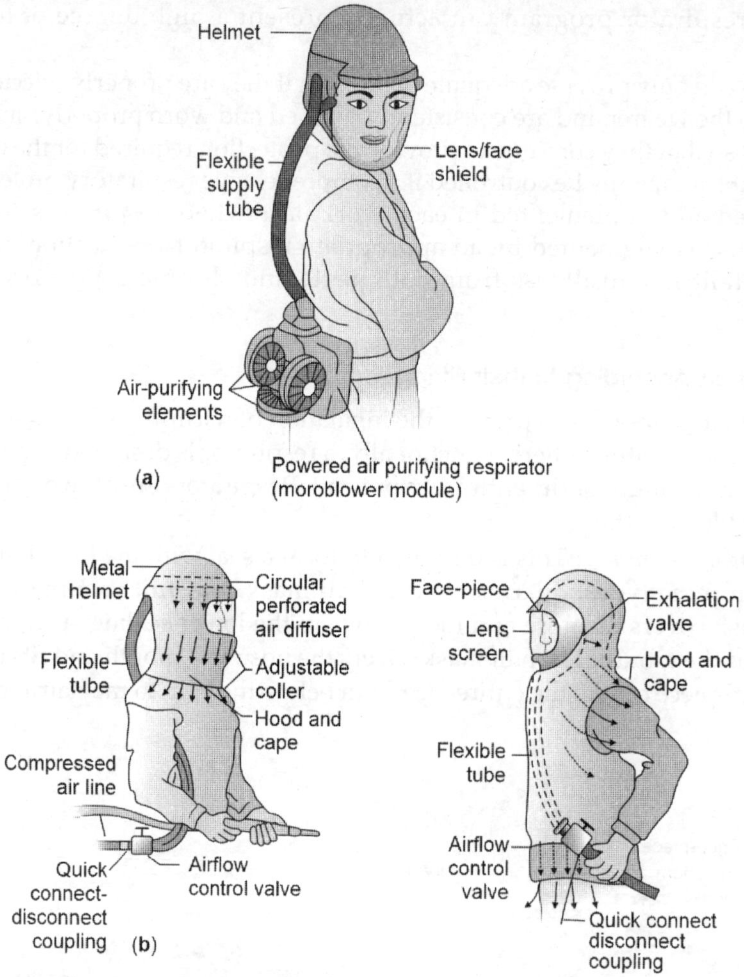

Fig. 4.3: A. Loose-fitting face-piece; B. Abrasive blasting respirator

2. *The loose-fitting respirator*: This has a respiratory inlet covering that is designed to form a partial seal with the face. These include loose-fitting face-pieces, as well as hoods, helmets, blouses, or full suits, all of which cover the head completely (Fig. 4.3a). The best known loose-fitting respirator is the supplied air hood used by the abrasive blaster (Fig. 4.3b). The hood covers the head, neck and upper torso, and usually includes a neck cuff. Air is delivered by a compressor through a hose leading into the hood. Because the hood is not tight-fitting, it is important that sufficient air is provided to maintain a slight positive-pressure inside the hood relative to the environment immediately outside the hood. In this way, an outward flow of air from the respirator will prevent contaminants from entering the hood.

Legal Requirement

In the (Indian) Factories Act, 1948 there are specific provisions for providing the personal protect equipment to the workers who are exposed to unsafe and unhealthy environment. The provisions of law relating to use of personal protective equipment in different operations and processes are framed in such a spirit that the workers working on the operations and in processes are protected against possible hazards. It is also the intention of the law that the personal protective equipment shall be of such type and made of such materials that withstand to such specific hazards for which it is actually being used.

Need for Respiratory PPE

In industry it may be possible to substitute a dangerous substance with a safer substance, isolate the process, to have automatic and mechanical handling of the substance or to have controlled ventilation of the process or to plan and arrange operation that personal protective equipment is not necessary, but sometimes it may not be possible to introduce such measures or there might be a breakdown in the plant or in the control measure. Under such circumstances it will become necessary to use personal protective equipment. It must be borne in mind the personal protective equipment does not eliminate a hazard. These devices designed to interpose an effective barrier between a person and harmful objects, substances or deviations.

Requirement of Respiratory Personal Protective Equipment

Requirements of suitable personal protective equipment can be listed as under:

1. Nature of the hazard
2. Severity of the hazard
3. Type of contaminant
4. Concentration of the contaminants
5. Duration of work
6. Location of the contaminated area with respect to a source of respirable air
7. Expected activity of the wearer
8. Operating characteristic and limitations of the equipment
9. Reliability of the equipment
10. Acceptance of the wearer
11. Cost of equipment.

Respiratory Hazards

Airborne hazards may result from either an oxygen deficient atmosphere or breathing air contaminated with toxic particles, vapors, gases, fumes or mist. The proper selection and use of a respirator depend on an initial determination of the concentration of the hazard or hazards present in the workplace, or the presence of an oxygen deficient atmosphere (Fig. 4.4). Airborne hazards generally fall into the following basic categories:

1. *Dusts:* Particles that are formed or generated from solid organic or inorganic materials by reducing their size through mechanical processes, such as crushing, grinding, drilling, abrading, or blasting.
2. *Fumes:* Particles formed when a volatilized solid, such as metal, condenses in cool air. This physical change is often accompanied by a chemical reaction, such as oxidation, e.g. lead oxide fumes from smelting, and iron oxide fumes from arc-welding. A fume can also be formed when a material such as magnesium metal is burned or when welding or gas cutting is done on galvanized metal.
3. *Mists:* A mist is formed when a finely divided liquid is suspended in the air. These suspended liquid droplets can be generated by condensation from the gaseous to the

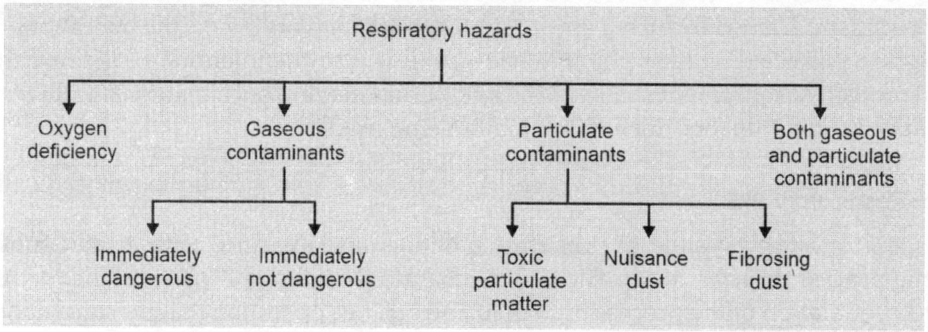

Fig. 4.4: Types of respiratory hazards

liquid state or by breaking up a liquid into a dispersed state, such as by splashing or atomizing, e.g. the oil mist produced during cutting and grinding operations, paint spray mist from spraying operations, and the condensation of water vapor to form a fog or rain.

4. *Gases:* Gases are formless fluids that occupy the space or enclosure and which can be changed to the liquid or solid state only by the combined effect of increased pressure and decreased temperature, e.g. welding gases, such as acetylene, nitrogen, helium and argon; and carbon monoxide generated from the operation of internal combustion engines. Another example is hydrogen sulfide, which is formed wherever there is decomposition of materials containing sulfur under reducing conditions.
5. *Vapors:* Vapors are the gaseous form of substances that are normally in the solid or liquid state at room temperature and pressure. They are formed by evaporation from a liquid or solid, and can be found where parts cleaning and painting takes place and where solvents are used.
6. *Smoke:* Smoke consists of carbon or soot particles resulting from the incomplete combustion of carbonaceous materials such as coal or oil. Smoke usually contains droplets as well as dry particles. When smoke is mixed with fog, it is known as smog.

Classification of Hazards

Type of hazards to which a worker is exposed is the basis of selection of the right type of respiratory protective equipment. The hazards may be classified as under:

1. *Oxygen deficiency*: An oxygen deficient atmosphere has oxygen content below 19.5% by volume. Atmosphere in confined spaces, such as vast tanks, holds of the ships, storage tanks, process vessels, sewers, septic tanks, underground utility tunnels, manholes, pits, etc. may contain air with oxygen content much lower than the normal (21% by volume). This may be due to dilution or displacement of the air by other gases or vapors or because of loss of oxygen due to decay of organic matter, chemical reaction and natural oxidation over a long period of time. A person breathing air with oxygen content of 16% or less may exhibit symptoms ranging from increased rate of breathing, acceleration of pulse rate to unconsciousness and death. Such oxygen deficiency conditions can easily be detected as the flame of a safety lamp will be extinguished in such atmosphere. The respiratory protective equipment, in such conditions, should either supply normal air or oxygen to the wearer.
2. *Gaseous contaminants*: These may be toxic or inert gases. The toxic gases may produce harmful effect even if they are present in relatively low concentrations. The inert gases

produce undesirable effects primarily by displacement of oxygen. Gaseous contaminants are two types:

i. *Gaseous contaminants immediately dangerous to life*: These contaminants are gases present in concentrations that would endanger life of a worker breathing them even for a short period of time. In other words, a gas is immediately dangerous to life if it is present in higher concentration. Where it is not possible to determine the extent of concentration or the kind of gas is not known, all gases should be considered as immediately dangerous to life.

ii. *Gaseous contaminants not immediately dangerous to life*: These contaminants are gases present in concentration that could be breathed by a worker for a short time without endangering his life but which may cause possible injury after a prolonged single expose or repeated short exposure. But even after the concentration of the contaminant is known, no exact formula can be applied to determine if the contaminant is immediately dangerous to life or not.

3. *Particulate contaminants (dusts, fumes, smokes, mists, fogs):* Majority of particulate contaminants are not immediately dangerous to life. They may be solid, liquid, or a combination of solid and liquid and may be classified into three broad groups:

i. *Toxic particulate contaminants*: These when inhaled may pass from the lungs into the bloodstream and are then carried to the various parts of the body, the effect may be chemical irritation, systemic poisoning or allergic reactions. Common contaminants in this group are antimony, arsenic, cadmium, chronic acid and chromates, lead and manganese.

ii. *Fibrosis-producing dusts*: These dusts do not pass into the bloodstream but remain in the lungs and may cause pulmonary impairment. The common examples under this group are asbestos, coal, bauxite and free silica.

iii. *Nuisance dust*: These may dissolve and pass directly into the bloodstream or may remain in the lungs neither producing local or systemic effects. In contrast to fibrogenic dusts which cause scar tissue in lungs when inhaled in excess amounts, so-called 'nuisance' dust have a long history little adverse effect on lungs and do not produce significant organic disease or toxic effect when exposures are kept under reasonable control. The nuisance dusts have also been called (biologically) 'inert' dusts, but the later term is inappropriate to the extent that there is no dust which does not evoke some cellular response in the lung when inhaled in sufficient amount. However, the lung-tissue reaction caused by inhalation of nuisance dusts has the following characteristics:

a. The architecture of the air spaces remains intact.

b. Collagen (scar tissue) is not form to a significant extent.

c. The tissue reaction is potentially reversible. Excessive concentrations of nuisance dusts in the workroom air may seriously reduce visibility, may cause unpleasant deposits in the eyes, ears, and nasal passages (i.e. Portland cement dust, chalk dust) or cause injury to the skin or mucous membranes by the chemical or mechanical action per se or by the rigorous skin cleaning procedures necessary for their removal. A threshold limit of 10 mg/m^3 of total dust $<1\%$ quartz are recommended for substances in these categories and for which no specific threshold limits have been assigned.

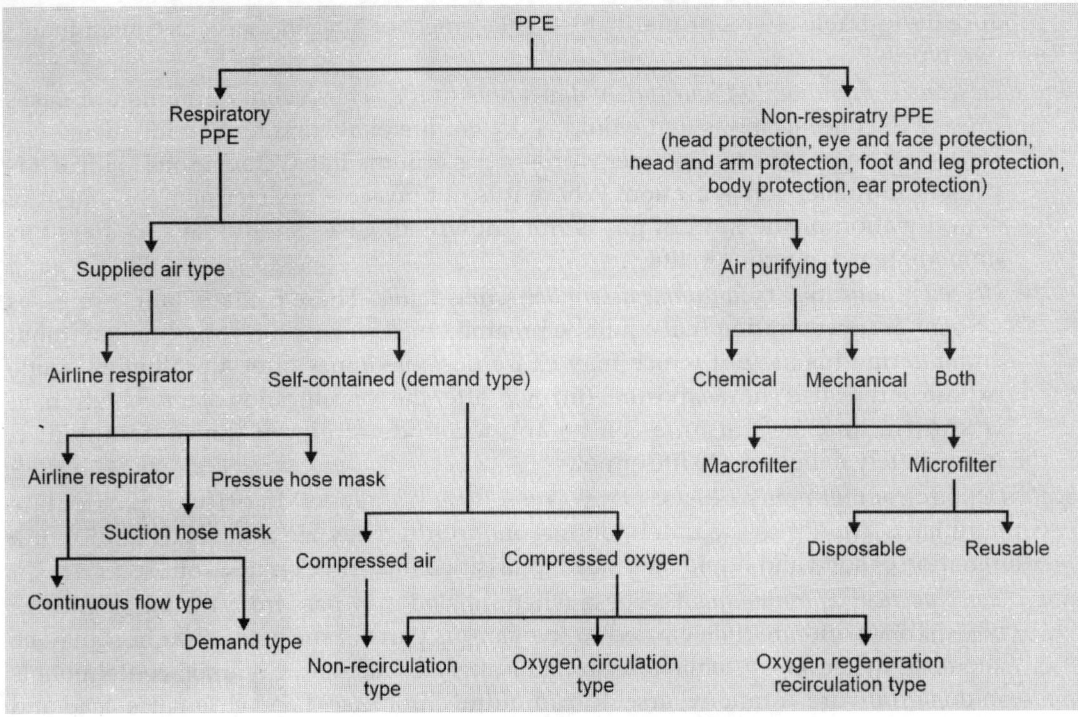

Fig. 4.5: Types of respiratory PPE

4. Combination of gaseous and particulate contaminants: The gaseous and particulate contaminants may be entirely of different substances like carbon-monoxide and oxides of nitrogen produced by blasting and the dust from the blasted material or they may be the same substances in liquid and vapor form like volatile liquids.

Types of Respiratory PPE (Fig. 4.5)

Supplied Air type

1. *Airline respirator*: Airline respirator consists of a face-piece (half or full mask or a loose-fitting helmet of hood to which air is supplied through a small diameter hose (Fig. 4.6). Airline respirators are of three types:
   a. Airline respirators: It may be a continuous flow type or demand type:
      i. *Continuous flow type*: Air is supplied continuously to the face-piece helmet or hood. Exhaled air or the excess air entering the face-piece escapes to the atmosphere. Air supplied should be at least 110 liters of air per minute to enter the face-piece at least 170 liters per minute to enter the helmet or hood.
      ii. *Demand type*: Respiratory air is supplied to a face-piece when the wearer inhales and the rate is governed by his volume rate of breathing. Air from an air

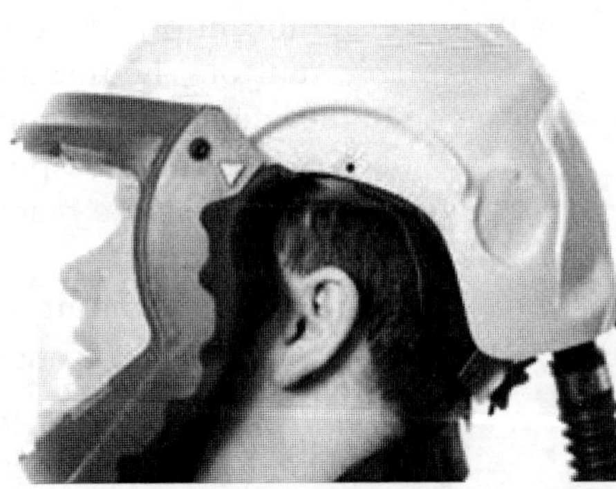

Fig. 4.6: Airline respirator

compressor cylinder of composed air is supplied to the face-piece through a demand valve which is situated by the slight negative pressure created when the wearer inhales. On exhalation the demand valve closes and exhaled air escapes to the surrounding atmosphere through exhalation valve. Helmets or hoods are not used with demand type respiratory.

Airline respirators provide protection so long as the air supply is maintained but the wearer's travel is restricted by the length of the air supply hose. Care should be taken to ensure that the air supply is not contaminated and is free from objectionable odors, oil or water mist and rust particles from the supply line.

b. *Suction hose mask:* It consists of a full face-piece connected to a large diameter flexible hose. The wearer draws in air by his own breathing effort, the hose is attached to the wearer's body by a suitable safety harness with safety line and the air inlet end of the hose is provided with a filter arrest particulate matter. Air can be drawn in by inspiratory effort of the wear up to 30 ft. length of the hose.

c. *Pressure hose mask*: This hose mask is similar to suction hose mask except that the air is forced through a large diameter hose by a hand or motor-operated blower. The blower is to be operated continuously while the mask is in use.

2. *Self-contained compressed air or oxygen breathing apparatus:* This is equipment by means of which wearer obtains respirable air or oxygen from compressed air or oxygen cylinder which is an integral part of the apparatus. In self-contained breathing apparatus, when the wearer inhales the quantity of air or oxygen admitted is governed by his breathing. The wearer exhaled air escapes to the surrounding atmosphere (*non-recirculating type*). In compressed oxygen cylinder *re-circulating type* breathing apparatus, high pressure oxygen from the cylinder passes through a pressure reducing and regulating valve into a breathing bag. The wearer inhales this oxygen through a one-way breathing valve and his exhaled breath passes into a canister containing chemicals to absorb exhaled carbon dioxide and moisture and then through a cooler into the same breathing bag. Oxygen enters the breathing bag from the supply cylinder only when the volume of gas in the bag has decreased sufficiently to allow the supply valve to open (Fig. 4.7)

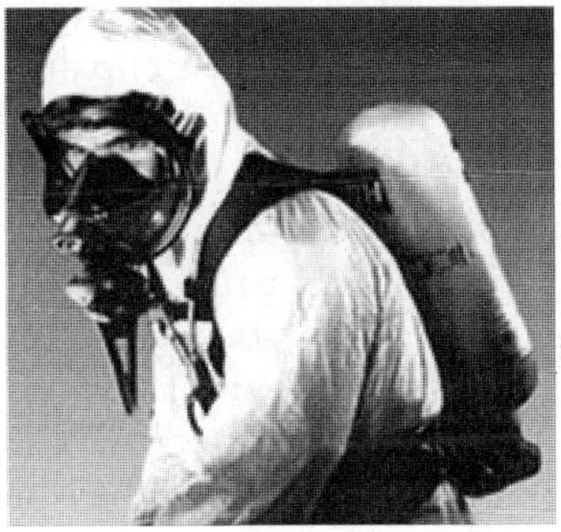

Fig. 4.7: Self-contained breathing apparatus

From respiratory point of view, self-contained breathing apparatus has no limitation as to the concentration of the gas or deficiency in the surrounding atmosphere but other factors may limit the activities. Many gases are very irritating to the skin and many can be absorbed in dangerous amounts through the unbroken skin.

Oxygen regenerating recirculating type: In this apparatus moisture content from the wearer's exhaled breath reacts with granular chemical in a canister to liberate oxygen. Also, the exhaled carbon dioxide is absorbed by the chemicals in the canister. This oxygen enters the breathing bag from which the wearer inhales through a corrugated breathing tube connecting the bag to the face-piece.

Air Purifying Respirators

1. *Chemical respirators:* These are three types:
   a. *Canister-gas mask*: This consists of a canister, containing appropriate chemical, a full face-piece and body harness to hold the canister in place on the body of the wearer. Air is drawn through the canister by the wearer and during its passage through the canister the contaminant present in the incoming air is absorbed in the chemical. The canisters are designed for specific gases. The canister gas mask can only be used in atmosphere not deficient in oxygen and not containing >2% by volume of most toxic gases. Also, the life of the canister will depend upon the type of canister, the concentration of gas and activity of the wearer (Fig. 4.8).

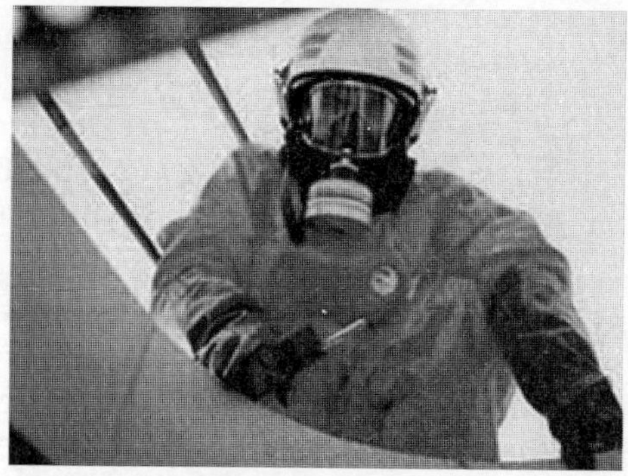

Fig. 4.8: Canister

   b. *Cartridge*: Like canister gas mask, chemical carriage respiratory provides respiratory protection for a period that depends on the type of cartridge used, the concentration of the gas or vapor, and the wearer's activity. It is recommended for low concentration gases and vapors (maximum of 0.1% of organic vapor).
   c. *Self-rescue type respirators*: This is designed to provide the greatest possible respiratory protection consistent with practicability of carrying the device at all times so that it is always available for use during escape. It consists of a small filter element, a mouth-piece, a nose clip and means of carry in conveniently on the body, the filter elements are similar to chemical cartridge. The extent of protection aforesaid is between that provided by canister gas mask and that prcvided by chemical cartridge respirator.
2. *Mechanical filter respirators:* These remove particulate matter from the inspired air which passes through a filter. These filters may be of the single use or re-usable type. If these respirators are used in heavy concentration of particulate matter, the filter will be clogged with dust particulate too quickly and they may have to be replaced every now and then. Microfilters are special filter designed to arrest ultra-microscopic size of dust particles and these are used where external fine dust are encountered (Fig. 4.9).
3. *Combination of chemical and mechanical filter respirators:* They remove toxic gases and vapors and particulate matter from inspired air. Example of their use is in spray painting work.

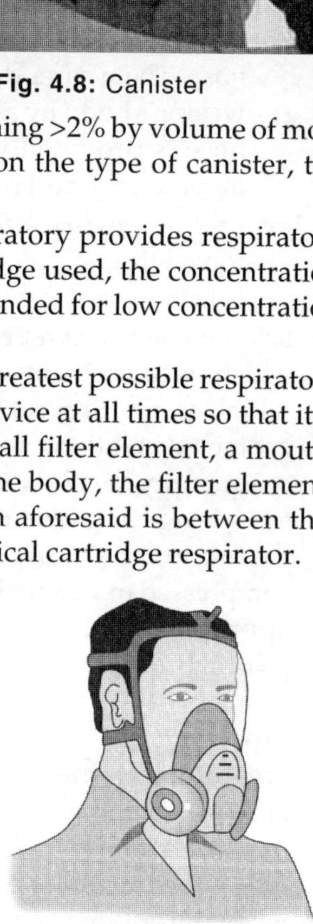

Fig. 4.9: Respiratory protection with filtration full mask

Respiratory Protection Program

Standard

Whenever respirators are required to be worn, a written respiratory protection program must be developed and implemented in accordance with OSHA's respiratory standard, 29 CRF 1910, 314. Additional program requirements may be found in the standards that regulate the hazards to which the employee is exposed. Because the workplaces differ substantially, each program must be tailored to the specific conditions of the workplace. The program must consist of worksite-specific procedures governing the selection, use and care of respirators.

The program must be updated as often as necessary to reflect changes in workplace conditions and respirator use.

Worksite-specific Procedure

This must contain all the information needed to maintain an effective respirator program to meet the user's individual requirements. These procedures are a set of step-by-step instructions written so that the task (i.e. respirator use, fit testing procedures, cleaning and storage, etc.) can be performed by all personnel in a uniform and consistent way, while supplying the maximum protection for workers who use respirators in the workplace. The employer must anticipate both the routine and non-routine use of respirators, as well as any possible emergency use based on the conditions in the workplace in which they are to be used. Worksite-specific procedure must be written so as to be useful to those who are directly involved in the respirator program: the program administrator, those fitting the respirators and training the workers, respirators maintenance workers, and the supervisors responsible for overseeing respirator use on the job.

Administration

In addition, the respirator standard requires the respiratory protection program be administered by one qualified individual to ensure that the integrity of the respiratory protection program is maintained through the continuous oversight of one responsible person. The program administrator must be qualified by appropriate training and/or experience in the proper selection. Use and maintenance of respirators, be responsible for implementing the respiratory protection program, and conduct regular evaluations of the program's effectiveness.

Elements

The respiratory protection program must cover the following basic elements, as applicable:

1. Procedure for selecting respirators for use in the workplace.
2. Medical evaluations of employees required to use respirators.
3. Fit testing procedures for tight-fitting respirators.
4. Use of respirators in routine and reasonably foreseeable emergency situations.
5. Procedures and schedules for cleaning, disinfecting, storing, inspecting, repairing, and otherwise maintaining respirators.
6. Procedures to ensure adequate air quality, quantity, and flow of breathing air for atmosphere-supplying respirators.
7. Training of employees in the respiratory hazards to which they are potentially exposed.
8. Training of employees in proper use of respirators, including putting on and removing them, any limitations on their use, and maintenance procedures.
9. Procedures for regularly evaluating the effectiveness of the program.

Selection of Respirator

Respiratory selection requires correctly matching the respirator with the hazard, the degree of hazard and the user. The respirator selected must be adequate to effectively reduce the exposure of the respirator user under all conditions of use, including reasonably foreseeable emergency situations. Proper respirator selection involves choosing a device that fully protects the worker from the respiratory hazards to which he or she may be exposed and permits the worker to perform the job with the least amount of physical burden. The following factors should be considered:

a. *Nature of the hazard, and the physical and chemical properties of the contaminant*: Nature of the hazard, whether it is in the form of gas, dust, organic vapor, fume, mist or oxygen deficiency or any combination of the hazards, needs to be taken into account. The physical and chemical properties of the contaminant that affect respirator selection, and the selection of the respirator components, such as cartridges, canisters, and filters must also be considered. Physical properties include such factors as particle size for dusts, vapor pressure for gases and vapors. Chemical properties of the air contaminant that affect breakthrough times, and the ability of the filter material to remove, or absorb the contaminant must also be considered.
b. *Concentration of the contaminant*: Sampling and analysis of the workplace air determines what degree of exposure is occurring, and thus what degree of protection is required. Where such sampling and analysis have been done, the results are to be used as a point of comparison with the occupational exposure level, i.e. to determine how much the concentration must be lowered by the respirator to reduce employee exposure to a safe level.
c. *Relevant permissible exposure limit or other occupational exposure limit*: Respirators selected must be capable of protecting against overexposure by reducing and maintaining exposure to or below the relevant exposure limit. In addition to OSHA limits, employers should refer to the ACGIH (American Conference of Governmental Industrial Hygienists) recommended Threshold Limit Values (TLV's), the NIOSH (National Institute for Occupational Safety and Health) Recommended Exposure Limits (REL's), or other occupational exposure limits.
d. *Nature of the work operation or process*: The type of job operation, the equipment or tools that will be used, and any motion or travel the job requires can influence the type of respirator selected, particularly when supplied-air respirators, which require a connection to a clean air source, are used.
e. *Time period the respirator is worn*: The employer must also consider the period of time during which the respirator will be used by employees during a work shift. Breakthrough times for different chemicals can vary greatly, and are dependent on the concentrations of contaminants in the workplace air, patterns of respirator used, and environmental factors including temperature and humidity. A respirator that provides adequate protection for one chemical may be inadequate for another chemical with a different breakthrough time. In addition, employees wearing respirators for longer periods of time may need respirators that impose the minimum possible physical burden.
f. *Work activities and physical/psychological stress*: Work activities of employees while wearing respirators are also a factor. Heavy work that is physically draining may affect an employee's capability of wearing certain types of respirators. Temperature and humidity conditions in the workplace may also affect the physical/psychological stress level associated with wearing a respirator, as well as the effectiveness of respirator filters and cartridges. These types of factors must be assessed in selecting the appropriate equipment for a particular work situation.
g. *Fit testing*: Some employees may be unable to achieve an adequate fit with certain respirator models or a particular type of respirator, such as half-mask air-purifying respirator, so an alternative respirator model with an adequate fit or other type of respirator that provides adequate protection must be used. Therefore, it is necessary for

employers to provide a sufficient number of respirator models and sizes from which employees can choose an acceptable respirator that fit correctly.

h. *Physical characteristics, functional capabilities and limitations of respirators*: The last category of information to be considered when selecting respiratory protection is the physical characteristics, functional capabilities, and limitation of the respiratory protection equipment itself. Respirators selected must not impair the worker's vision, hearing, communication, and physical movement necessary to perform jobs safely. For example, airline respirators should not be used by mobile employees around moving machinery to avoid entanglement of the respirator in the equipment.
i. Severity of the hazard.
j. Types of contaminants.
k. Location of the contaminated area with respect to a source of respirable air.

Atmosphere Requiring Highest Level of Protection

For atmospheres that are immediately dangerous to life and health (IDLH), the highest level of respiratory protection and reliability is required. These atmospheres, by definition, are the most dangerous environments in which respirators are used. In these atmospheres, there is no tolerance for respirator's failure. Consequently, only the following respirators must be provided and used: full-face-piece pressure demand self-contained breathing apparatus (SCBA) certified for a minimum service life of thirty minutes, or a combination full face-piece pressure demand supplied-air respirator (SAR) with an auxiliary self-contained air supply.

Atmospheres are IDLH when they pose an immediate threat to life, would cause irreversible adverse health effects, or would interfere with an individual's ability to escape from a dangerous atmosphere. Care must be exercise in these situations since failure of the respirator to provide the appropriate protection may result in serious injury or death. Consequently, the employer must develop and implement specific procedures for the use of respirators in IDLH atmospheres that include the following provisions:

1. At least one employee (referred to as 'standby employee') is to be located outside the IDLH atmosphere and maintain visual, voice, or signal line communication with the employee(s) in the IDLH atmosphere.
2. The standby employee(s) located outside the IDLH atmosphere must be trained and equipped to provide effective emergency rescue.
3. The employer or authorized designee is to be notified before the standby employee(s) enter the IDLH atmosphere to provide emergency rescue.
4. The employer or authorized designee, once notified to such entry, must provide the necessary assistance appropriate to the situation.
5. Standby employee(s) must be equipped with pressure demand or other positive pressure SCBA or a pressure demand or other positive pressure supplied-air respirator with auxiliary SCBA.
6. Standby employee(s) must be equipped with appropriate retrieval equipment for lifting or removing the employee from the hazardous atmosphere, or, when such retrieval equipment cannot be used because it would increase the overall risk resulting from entry, ensure that equivalent provision for rescue have been made.

Care of Respirator

The OSHA standard requires that employers provide each respirator user with a respirator that is clean, sanitary, and in good working order. These requirements are a vital part of any successful respiratory protection program. To ensure that the respirator remains serviceable and delivers effective protection, a maintenance program must be in place prior to respirator use. The OSHA respirator standard strongly emphasizes the important of a good maintenance program, but permits its tailoring to the type of facilities, working conditions, and hazards involved. However, all programs are required to include at least:

1. Cleaning and disinfecting procedures.
2. Proper storage.
3. Regular inspections for defects (including leak check).
4. Repair methods.

In addition to the OSHA requirements, the manufacturer's instructions for inspection, cleaning, and maintenance of respirators should be consulted to ensure that the respirator continues to function properly. A proper maintenance program ensures that the worker's respirator remains as effective as when it was new.

Instructions in the use of respirators, among other thing, should include the following aspects:

a. Why it is to be used
b. How it is to be used
c. Checking that it is in good operating condition
d. Fitting or respirator
e. Proper use and maintenance of the respirator.

Respiratory protective equipment testing facilities are available at Central Labour Institute, Directorate General Factory Advice Service and Labour Institutes, Ministry of Labour and Employment, Government of India, Sion, Mumbai-400022. Realizing the needs and problems faced by the manufacturers in the country, a respirator testing laboratory (RTL) and a non-respiratory testing laboratory (NRTL) have been established in the Central Labour Institute at Mumbai. This laboratory undertakes the testing of indigenously manufactured respiratory protective devices under prescribed test conditions. This laboratory is equipped with facilities for testing breathing resistance, face-place leakage, and exhalation valve leakage, filtration efficiency against a standard dust, test of canisters and cartridges against known concentration of specific gases or vapor. The performance standards suggested in the USA are generally followed. This laboratory presently carries out the above tests and submits factual performance reports to the manufacturers. Non-respiratory PPE testing facilities (like safety shoe, helmet, etc.) are available there.

Medical Evaluation Program

Persons assigned to task that require the use of a respirator must be physically able to perform the work while using the respirator. Accordingly, employers have the responsibility of ensuring that employees are medically fit to tolerate the physical and psychological stress imposed by respirator use, as well as the physical stress originating from job and workplace conditions. Employees must be medically evaluated and found eligible to wear the respirator selected for their use prior to fit testing or first-time use of the respirator in the workplace.

The purpose of medical evaluation program is to determine if employees can tolerate the physiological burden associated with respirator use, including, the burden imposed by the respirator itself (e.g. its weight and breathing resistance during both normal operation and under conditions of filter, canister, or cartridge overload); musculoskeletal stress (e.g. when the respirator to be worn is a SCBA); limitation of auditory, visual, and olfactory sensations;

and isolations from the workplace environment. Since certain jobs and workplace conditions in which a respirator is used can also impose a physiological burden to the user, the medical evaluation must also consider the following factors: type and the weight of the respirator to be worn, duration and frequency of respirator use; expected physical work effort; use of protective clothing and equipment to be worn; and temperature and humidity extremes that may be encountered.

The medical evaluation is designed to identify general medical conditions that place employees who use respirators at risk of serious medical consequences. Medical conditions known to compromise an employee's ability to tolerate respirator-, job-, workplace-related physiological stress include: Cardiovascular and respiratory diseases (e.g. history of high blood pressure, angina, heart attack, cardiac arrhythmias, stroke, asthma, chronic bronchitis, emphysema); reduced pulmonary function caused by the other factors (e.g. smoking or prior exposure to the respiratory hazards), neurological or musculoskeletal disorders (e.g. ringing of the ears, epilepsy, lower back pain); impaired sensory function (e.g. perforation ear drums, reduced or absent ability to smell); and psychological disorders (e.g. claustrophobia and severe anxiety).

Training and Information

a. Employee training is an important part of the respiratory protection program and is essential for correct respirator use. The OSHA respiratory protection standard requires employers to provide training before employee uses a respirator in the workplace. For the training to be effective, the training information must be comprehensive and presented in an understandable way.
b. Employers should develop training program based on the employees' educational level and language background. Such an approach will ensure that all employees receive training that enables them maximize the effectiveness of the respirators they use. As a result of this training, the employee will be able to understand the operation of the respirator and demonstrate the ability to properly use the respirator.
c. Employees' training must include a discussion of why the use of the respirator is necessary. Such training would address the identification of the hazards involved, the extent of employee exposures to those hazards, and the potential health effects of such exposures.
d. Information regarding the consequences of improper fit, usages, or maintenance on respirator effectiveness must also be provided to employees. Inadequate attention of any of these program elements would obviously defeat the effectiveness of the respirator. Proper fit, usage, and maintenance of respirators are critical to ensure employee protection.
e. Employees must be provided with an explanation of the limitations and capabilities of the respirator selected for employee use. A discussion of the limitations and capabilities of respirator must address how the respirator operates. This training would include, e.g. an explanation of how the respirator provides protection by either filtering the air, absorbing the vapor or gas, or providing clean air from an uncontaminated source. Where appropriate, it should include limitations on the use of the equipment, such as prohibitions against using an air-purifying respirator in IDLH atmospheres and an explanation of why such a respirator should not be used in these situations.

f. Employees must also know how to use the respirator effectively in emergency situations, including those in which the respirator malfunctions. Comprehensive training is necessary where respirators are used in IDLH situations, including oxygen-deficient atmospheres such as those that occur in fire-fighting, rescue operations and confined-area entry.
g. Training must include the procedures for inspecting the respirator, checking the fit and respirator seal. Employees must be capable of recognizing any problems that may threaten the continued protective capability of the respirator.
h. Instruction must be given regarding the proper procedures for maintenance and storage of respirators.

The training program must also provide employees with medical information that is sufficient for them to recognize the signs and symptoms of medical conditions that may limit or prevent the effective use of respirator.

Chapter

5

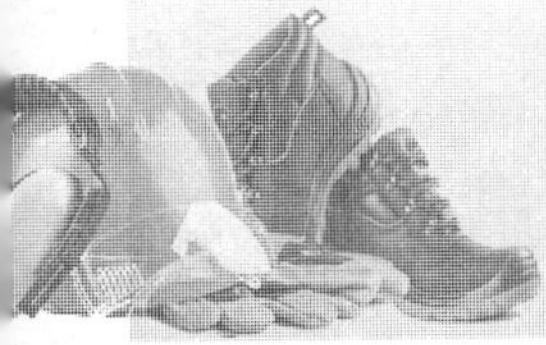

First-Aid

First-aid is the immediate and temporary care given to a person in case of injury or sudden illness and the purpose of first aid is to preserve life, assist recovery, prevent aggravation and minimize complication at the later dates with the help of such material as may be available.

Scope of First Aid

1. To determine the nature of the case of requiring attention for efficient treatment.
2. To decide on the character and extent of each case requiring treatment.
3. To determine the extent of treatment to be given.
4. To apply the most suited treatment in the circumstances until medical aid is available.
5. To arrange for the transportation of the case to the home or suitable place or hospital.

Principle of First Aid

1. Maintenance of oxygen exchange, i.e. breathing.
2. Control of hemorrhage/bleeding.
3. Prevention of shock.
4. Splinting of fractures for broken bone.
5. Evaluation of any other condition like burn, etc.
6. Application of appropriate first aid.

Rules of First Aid

1. Do first thing first—quickly, quietly and without panic.
2. Artificial respiration—if breathing has stopped.
3. Arrest bleeding.
4. Prevent or treat shock.
5. Do not attempt too much.
6. Reassure the casualty.
7. Do not allow people to crowd around.
8. Remove unnecessary clothing.
9. Arrange for transportation to hospital for proper treatment.

Aim of First Aid

1. To promote recovery.
2. To preserve life.
3. To prevent worsening of casualty's conditions.
4. Arrange transportation, if necessary.

The first aider should:

1. Be careful.
2. Think clearly.
3. Act quickly.
4. Be calm and cool.
5. Be confident.
6. Not be excited.
7. Inform ambulance/doctor immediately.
8. Give first aid methodically.
9. Assure casualty.

First Aid Leaflet (Instruction for Handling Emergencies)

Shock

1. Lay the patient on his back.
2. Stop bleeding if any.
3. Relieve pain by supporting injured part.
4. Keep the patient comfortable. Do not cause sweating.
5. Fluids may be given in small amounts unless the patient is nauseated, unconscious, likely to be operated on, or has an abdominal wound.
6. Reassure and cheer up the patient.

Wounds

1. Stop the bleeding by anyone of the following methods:
   a. Direct pressure.
   b. Direct finger pressure into the wound in cases of larger bleeding wounds.
   c. Tourniquet (seldom needed)—use only as a last resort.
2. Avoid touching the wound with hands or unsterile material.
3. Clean the wound with running water and surrounding area with soap or spirit with clean gauze washing away from the wound. Apply ready-made adhesive gauze, bandage or sterile gauze and roller bandage as needed.
4. Keep the patient quiet; raising the extremity if it is the bleeding part. Give no stimulants.
5. Never apply antiseptic ointment, lotion, or iodine or germicide to the wound.

Abdominal Wounds

1. No time must be lost in sending the patient to the hospital.
2. Keep the patient flat.
3. Give nothing by mouth.
4. Maintain warmth.
5. If intestines protrude from the wound do not attempt to touch or replace them.

6. Apply sterile dressing and binder.
7. Provide careful, immediate transportation to the hospital.

Eye Wounds

1. Removal may be attempted if foreign body is not embedded.
2. Do not apply oil or ointment.
3. If there is a foreign body embedded in the eyeball, send the worker immediately to the doctor after applying pad and loose bandage.

Chemical Burns of the Eyes

1. Immediately washing of the eye at least for fifteen minutes is of great importance.
2. Apply sterile bandage and send the worker immediately to the doctor.
3. Neutralizing agents or ointments should not be used.

Suffocation

1. Remove the patient from the source of danger.
2. Make a rapid examination to ensure that the air passages are free and to clean them if necessary.
3. Restore natural breathing by artificial respiration, if breathing has ceased.

Electric Shock

1. Remove the patient from the source of danger.
2. Make a rapid examination to ensure that the air passage is free and to clean them if necessary.
3. Restore natural breathing by artificial respiration, if breathing has ceased.

Insensibility

1. Send for a doctor if possible, pending his arrival.
2. Where the patient's face is pale, lay him flat and face downwards with his head turned to one side. If his face is flushed or blue, raise and support the head and shoulders.
3. Control any serious bleeding.
4. Loosen any tight clothing and let him have plenty of air.
5. Do not give anything by mouth.
6. If doctor is not available send the casualty to hospital.

Backbone (Spinal) Fracture

1. Transport on a rigid frame. This frame may be improvised by using available boards or a door.
2. The rigid frame may be placed on a stretcher for transportation.
3. If a firm frame cannot be improvised, transport patient on abdomen on a stretcher made of canvas or blanket.
4. In neck fracture cases it is much better to send the person to a doctor.

Burns

1. Act quickly.
2. Put the affected part in cold water.

3. Pour the water over burns that cannot be immersed (cold water relieves pain, reduces fluid loss).
4. Cover with a sterilized dressing.

Dealing with a Person whose Clothes have Caught Fire

1. Put out the flames by whatever means available. Pouring of water can solve the purpose. Pouring the cool water in the local burnt area can cause less damage to occur.
2. Do not allow the person to run about. This only fans the fire and makes the flame spread.
3. Hold a rug, blanket, coat or table cover in front of you, while approaching a man whose clothing have caught fire.
4. Lay him/her down quickly on the ground and wrap tightly with any thick piece of cloth, rug or coat. Smother the flame by gently rolling the casualty or by gently pats over the covering.

Fracture of Bone

1. Do not move the injured unless the life is in danger from other cause.
2. Deal with the Hemorrhage and breathing difficulties, if any.
3. Immobilize the fracture by the use of bandages using the injured body as support or by well-padded splint.
4. Immobilization should one point above and one point below. Remove the injured to the hospital.

Rescuing Person from Fire

1. In rescuing persons from a room which has caught fire, speed and clear thinking are required.
2. It should be remembered that clear air is at ground level. So, crawl along the floor to pull out a person who is lying unconscious or is disabled.
3. Have a wet handkerchief round your face when you will rescue the person.
4. If there is CO in the room, these precautions do not protect the rescuer from CO poisoning. Therefore, when there is fire in a close room, some amount of CO should always be present. You will have to take a quick action to avoid these hazards.
5. When there is fire in a room in which the doors and windows are closed, do not open them to let in air. The rush of air will increase the fire and it will burn more intensely.
6. If the person is unconscious on a bed, lay him/her on the floor and try to evacuate from the room as quick as possible.
7. After coming out of the room, if it is found that his/her heart beat and respiration have stopped, start cardiorespiratory resuscitation.
8. Do not give anything by mouth when the person is unconscious.
9. If the person has some burns in the body, he/she should be sent to the hospital with sterile conditions.

Who should be Admitted to Hospital with Burn

1. Adult with burns >20%.
2. Children with burns >10%.
3. Extreme of age.
4. Person with pre-existing chronic illness.

5. Person with diabetes.
6. Person with pre-existing cardiovascular diseases.
7. All electrical and chemical burn.
8. All burns involving important vital organs.
9. Burns associated with fractures and multiple injuries.

Calculation of the fire percentage of burn: Rule of nines

	Body area covered	*Percentage*
1.	Head and neck	9
2.	Right upper extremity	9
3.	Left upper extremity	9
4.	Front of the body	18 (9 + 9)
5.	Back of the body	18 (9 + 9)
6.	Right lower extremity	18 (9 + 9)
7.	Left lower extremity	18 (9 + 9)
8.	External genital organs	1
	Total body	100

Chapter

6

Pulmonary Function Test

At present, spirometry remains the most suitable screening test for routine industrial applications. The spirogram generally relates to morbidity as perceived by patient and physician when compared to other screening studies or tests for small airway disease. Pulmonary function test is necessary in pre-employment and periodical medical examinations for the protection of the workers in some industries (e.g. in the prevention of byssinosis where it is important to establish a baseline for future reference prior to exposure). Spirometry is effort dependent, and failure to obtain reproducible results usually reflects inadequate cooperation. However, it should be recognized that test failure (lack of reproducible results) may reflect ill health, making interpretation difficult. Additional pulmonary function tests are useful in clarifying confusion results and are best performed at a referral center when a ventilator impairment is suspected (Fig. 6.1). They are also of value in:

1. Determining the type and extent of any lung disease process.
2. Following the progression of the disease for changes in severity or in response to therapy,
3. Developing further understanding between the functional, radiological and pathological changes.
4. Legal and compensation purposes.

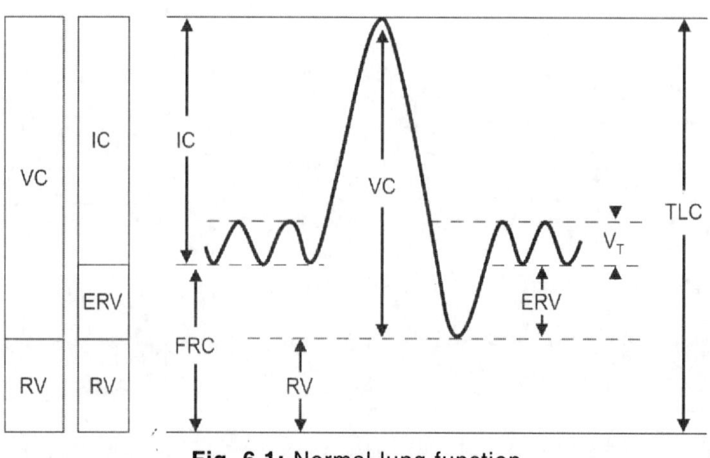

Fig. 6.1: Normal lung function

The variety of pulmonary functions is as follows (common measurements):

a. Tidal volume (V_T): The volume of gas inspired or expired during each respiratory cycle (normal value is 500 ml.).
b. Total lung capacity (TLC): The volume of gas contained in the lungs at the end of a maximum inspiration (normal value is 6 L)
c. Vital capacity (VC): The largest volume measured on complete expiration after deepest inspiration without forced or rapid effort (normal value is 4.8 L).
d. Inspiratory capacity (IC): The largest volume of gas that can be inspired from the resting expiratory level (normal value is 3.6 L).
e. Functional residual capacity (FRC): The volume of gas remaining in the lungs at the end-expiratory level (normal value is 2.4 L).
f. Expiratory reserve volume (ERV): The largest volume of gas that can be expired from the end-expiratory level (normal value is 1.2 L).
g. Inspiratory reserve volume (IRV): The largest volume of gas that can be inspired from the end-inspiratory level (normal value is 3.1 L).
h. Reserve volume (RV): The volume of gas remaining in the lungs at the end of maximum expiration (normal value is 1.2 L).

Indication of PFT

To determine the:

1. Presence of lung disease or abnormality of lung function.
2. Extent of abnormalities.
3. Extent of impairment caused by abnormal lung function.
4. Progression of disease.
5. Nature of physiologic disturbance.
6. Course of therapy for treatment of a particular lesion.

Variety of Pulmonary Functions (Common Measurements)

1. The vital capacity (VC) refers to the maximal volume of air that a patient can exhale after a maximal inspiration. If the exhalation is performed as forceful as possible, the volume is referred to as forced vital capacity (FVC). Changes in the vital capacity are more important than single determinations.
2. An estimate of the flow rates can be obtained by measuring the volume exhaled during the first second (FEV_1).
3. The maximal mid-expiratory flow rate measures the average flow rate during the middle half of the FVC and is referred to as the $FEF_{25-75\%}$ (forced expiratory flow between 25% and 75% of the FVC).
4. Obstructive index: $FEV_{1.0}$/FVC ratio—statement of $FEV_{1.0}$ as a percentage of the subjects actual FVC.
5. Restrictive index: Observed FVC/Pred. FVC ratio.
6. Peak expiratory flow rate (PEFR): Maximum flow rate attained at anytime during an FEV manoeuvre—it is usually measured by peak flow meter and the unit is liter per minute.

The residual volume (RV) can be determined by having the subject breathe through a spirometer circuit of constant volume for at least 7 minutes. By measuring the dilution of helium, which is used as a tracer gas, the residual volume of air remaining in the lungs at the completion of exhalation can be calculated. Alternative methods are available for determining the RV, including the open-circuit nitrogen washout method and body plethysmography. The total lung capacity (TLC) is the sum of the VC and the RV. An increase in the RV when accompanied by an increase in the RV/TLC ratio reflects pulmonary overdistention and probable air trapping. A reduction in the VC when accompanied by a decrease in the TLC reflects restrictive ventilatory impairment.

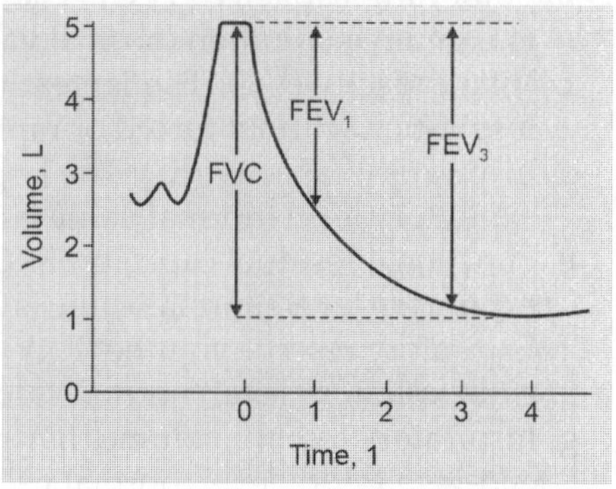

Fig. 6.2: Spirogram—volume time relationship

The maximum ventilator volume (MVV), formerly referred to as the maximum breathing capacity (MBC), is determined by measuring the volume of gas exchange 12 to 15 seconds of maximal voluntary hyperventilation. The test is dependent on motivation of the subject, muscles strength, fatigability, extent of air trapping and overall integrity of the spirometer (Figs 6.2 and 6.3).

The respiratory diffusion capacity (DL) is determined by measuring the amount of carbon monoxide that is transferred from the alveoli to hemoglobin in the pulmonary capillaries. Two methods are available—the single-breath method, during which the patient must hold his breath for 10 seconds and then exhale, and a steady-state method, which requires less cooperation of the patient but is more sensitive to imbalances of ventilation and perfusion. The DL is dependent on the surface area available for transfer of gas, the size of the pulmonary capillary bed, and the amount of hemoglobin present. The percent-predicted FEV_1, MVV and RV/TLC correlate closely with dyspnea in subjects with obstructive lung disease. With interstitial disease, a combination of <50% predicted for the FVC or 40% predicted for the DL is satisfactory criteria for the detection of subjects with disabling dyspnea.

Arterial blood gas (PaO_2 and $PaCO_2$) and PH often are normal at rest and become abnormal during exercise performed on a bicycle ergometer or on a treadmill. During exercise, the minute ventilation and oxygen consumption can be measured. The increased difference between alveolar and arterial oxygen tension [$(A - a)O_2$ gradient] at rest or after exercise often is an early indication of impaired gas exchange resulting from a mismatch in ventilation and perfusion. Pulmonary compliance refers to the distensibility of the lungs and can be calculated by measuring the change in intrathoracic volume for a given change in intrathoracic pressure. The pressure change is determined by the use of an esophageal balloon.

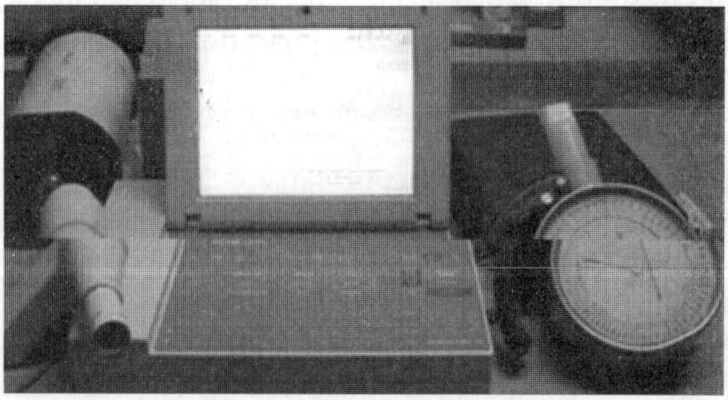

Fig. 6.3: Spirometer with calibrator and peak flow meter

Regional lung functions are done by fluoroscopy (mainly for movement of diaphragm and mediastinum), bronchospirometry, and radioisotope technique.

Differences between obstructive and restrictive lung disorders

Parameter	*Obstructive disorder*	*Restrictive disorder*
Total lung capacity (TLC)	↑	↓
Reserve volume (RV)	↑	↓
Vital capacity (VC), force vital capacity (FVC)	↓	↓
FEV_1/FVC%	↓	Normal/↑
RV/TLC%	↑	Normal
Resistance	↑	Normal
Compliance	↑	↓
Diffusion	Normal	↓
Arterial PO_2	↓	↓
Arterial PCO_2	↑	↓
Arterial PH	↓	Normal/↑

Interpretation of Pulmonary Function Test

- Normal test:
  - Observed FVC > 80% of predicted FVC
  - Observed FEV_1 > 75% of predicted FEV_1
- Obstructive impairment:
  - Observed FVC > 80% of predicted FVC
  - Observed FEV_1 < 75% of predicted FEV_1
- Restrictive impairment:
  - Observed FVC < 80% of predicted FVC
  - Observed FEV_1 > 75% of prêdicted FEV_1
- Combined (mixed) impairment:
  - Observed FVC < 80% of predicted FVC
  - Observed FEV_1 < 75% of predicted FEV_1

Predicted equations: Kamat SR, et al. equation:

Male	FVC	0.0503H – 0.0136A – 4.488
	FEV_1	0.0396H – 0.0212A – 3.130
	PEER	4.236H – 2.0981A – 109.5
Female	FVC	0.0370H – 0.0070A – 3.187
	FEV_1	0.0274H – 0.0103A – 1.995
	PEER	3.310H – 1.865A – 81.0

(H: height in cm; A: age in years)

Chapter

7

Audiometry Test

Industrial environments are seldom suitable for accurate tests of normal hearing, even though the medical facilities may be located in a relatively quit area. To determine the suitability of an area for audiometric testing, it is necessary to carry out environmental noise measurements during the noisiest anticipated conditions. From these studies, the degree of attenuation required to permit accurate threshold audiometry can be determined. In most instance, it will be cheaper and more satisfactory to purchase a prefabricated testing room (audiometry room/ booth) having sufficient attenuation to permit accurate threshold measurements under the worst conditions. To assure that audiogram taken in the plant prove acceptable technically, the program should be under the supervision of the medical director/incharge. In addition, the technician taking the measurement should be adequately trained. An industrial audiometric technician should be competent in obtaining medical and occupational exposure histories and measuring pure tone audiometric thresholds, when he observes abnormalities, he should refer the employee to a physician for examination. If the physician feels that special diagnostic tests are required, he may recommend that the employees receive diagnostic evaluation from an outside otologist or a hearing and speech center. Employee identification is important because it permits verification of the record and avoid duplication. This identification usually consists of the employee's name, age, sex, badge and staff number, etc. It is important that no two persons be identified by the same number and that individual numbers remain the same for each person during the period of study. A brief history of ear disease, previous noise exposure and family history of deafness should be included along with present occupational and para-occupational history should be included and a simple examination of the external canal and drum should be performed and recorded. If environmental noise measurement has been made in the area where the individual works, that location should be described as accurately and completely as possible. It is also desirable to record audiometric test conditions such as location and type of the test booth, manufacturer and type of audiometer, name of the examiner and method of procedure. Such factors as the day of work week, the hour of work day, and the interval between noise exposure and testing help to interpret the data. A hearing conservation program includes pre-placement, periodic (follow-up) and terminal audiogram for the exposed personnel. The specific interval between follow-up examinations will depend upon many factors including statutory requirement, the environmental noise exposure and the availability of the medical facilities. Where the sound pressure level in the working environment exceeds 85 dBA, follow-up threshold examinations should be instituted. The more the sound pressure level exceeds 85 dBA, the more urgent is the need for hearing conservation measure.

Measurement of hearing using electroacoustic devices is generally referred to as audiometry. Pure tone audiometry records the threshold at octave intervals covering the frequencies most commonly encountered in everyday life and in particular in everyday speech. The frequencies usually tested in the clinical setting are 125 Hz, 250 Hz, 500 Hz, 1 kHz, 2 kHz, 4 kHz and 8 kHz. In the medicolegal and compensation fields, 3 kHz are always tested and 6 kHz may be. Air and bone conduction thresholds are measured to establish the presence or absence of the conductive component of the overall hearing loss. Bone conduction thresholds are inaccurate above 3 kHz. Audiometry may be carried out by an audiometrician (manual audiometry). Important side issues include the calibration of the equipment, the acoustic requirements of the test area, instructions to the subject and the format and storing records.

The interpretation of individual audiograms is usually straightforward, particularly if a pre-placement/periodical audiogram is routinely performed and presented to the physician, who interprets changes in threshold levels which may have occurred between periodic audiometric tests. When differences of 10 dB or more are observed at >1 frequency at or below 2000 Hz or when differences are found to be of 20 dB or more at 4000 Hz or above, an explanation should be sought. If there is no medical explanation for such a change and if the situation suggests a noise factor, a study of all employees working in the noisy area may be desirable. When the number of employees is small, and when no engineering control of the noise hazard is readily available, the most practical control measure may be personal protection. Where statistically significant group difference has been demonstrated and correlated with noise exposure, it is easier to convinced management that the expensive engineering or personal control measures may be a good investment. However, to be effective, hearing conservation requires close supervision and medical follow-up as well as an educational program.

In evaluating the audiograms of employees from noisy environments, the possibility of temporary threshold shift should be recognized. Temporary threshold shift can be reduced or eliminated only by examining employees after they have been away from hazardous noise for 16 hours or more.

When permanent threshold shift is recognized in a large number of employees from a certain noisy department, management must be informed of the problem and its consequences. One or more control programs should be presented. When the permanent threshold shifts are limited to a small percent of exposed personnel who show progressive and significant changes in hearing threshold, a decision must be made as to whether the employees should be removed from the noisy exposure. Such a decision is very difficult and must be based on complete evaluation of the individual, the environment and the economic implications to both the individual and management. In the final analysis, the decision to remove an employee from a given noise exposure is a management decision but the evaluation and recommendation of the plant medical officer will weigh heavily upon it.

AUDIOLOGICAL CRITERIA

In addition to the quantitative criteria, workers showing variable or inconsistent responses or unusual hearing loss curves should be referred.

A. Baseline audiogram:

1. Average hearing level at 0.5, 1, 2, and 3 kHz >25 dB, in either ear.
2. Difference in average hearing level between the better and poorer ears of: (a) >10 dB at 0.5, 1, and 2 kHz, or (b) >20 dB at 3, 4, and 6 kHz.

B. Periodic audiogram: Change for the worse in average hearing level, in either ear, compared to the baseline audiogram of:

a. >10 dB at 0.5, 1, and 2 kHz
b. >20 dB at 3, 4, and 6 kHz.

AUDIOMETRY TEST PROCEDURE IN PURE TONE AUDIOMETER (Figs 7.1–7.3)

Air Conduction

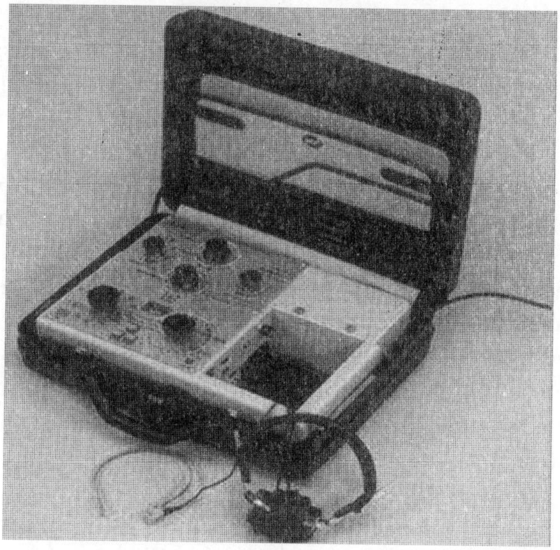

Fig. 7.1: Pure tone audiometer

The ear phone should be plugged into the jack socket on the side panel. The audiometer can be switched by operating the switch to 'on'. The mode switch can be turned to either 'right' or 'left' depending upon the ear to be tested. The frequency dial is then adjusted to the test frequency. It is advisable to start the test with 1000 Hz. Next go to each higher frequency up to 8000 Hz and then come back to 1000 Hz and retest at this frequency to find out the reliability of the worker's response. Thereafter, test the lower frequencies from 1000 Hz down. The intensity of the tone can be controlled by rotating the hearing loss attenuator (intensity dial), while testing each frequency, the intensity of the tone should be presented at a higher level to make the worker aware of the tone he is going to hear and then gradually bring down the intensity of the tone to his threshold. Threshold of hearing is the minimum audible intensity level for that particular frequency. Threshold is that level where the worker will give a 50% response (like, 'yes' – 'no' – 'yes', I can hear). The Audiogram thus plotted on a chart is called unmasked air conduction threshold.

Bone Conduction

The jack of the bone conduction vibrator is plugged into the socket on the side panel of the audiometer. The vibrator is placed on the Rt or Lt sided mastoid bone (back side of the pinna of ear). The mode switch is positioned to 'BC'. Bone conduction up to 4000 Hz only can be tested maximum. The testing procedure is the same as for air conduction. The audiogram thus plotted on a chart is called unmasked bone conduction threshold.

Symbols used: Right year—air conduction (AC) = O, bone conduction (BC) = >; Left ear—air conduction (AC) = X, bone conduction (BC) = <

Audiogram of ____________________

Address ____________________

__________ Date __________ Remarks

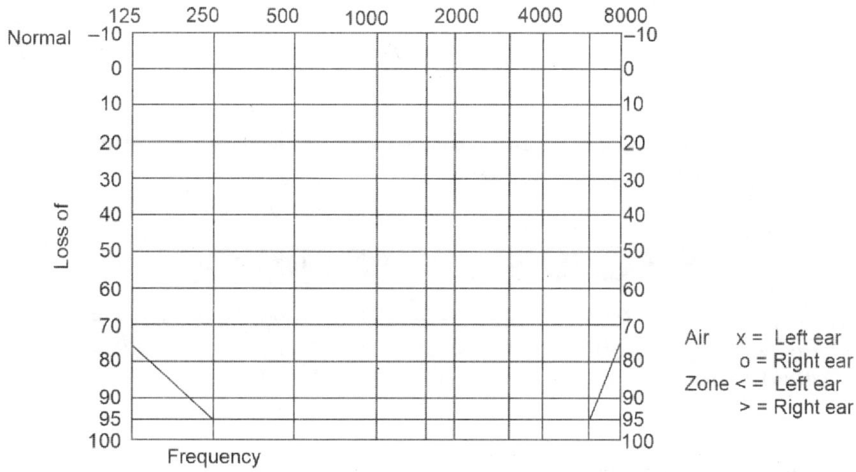

Fig. 7.2: Audiometry chart

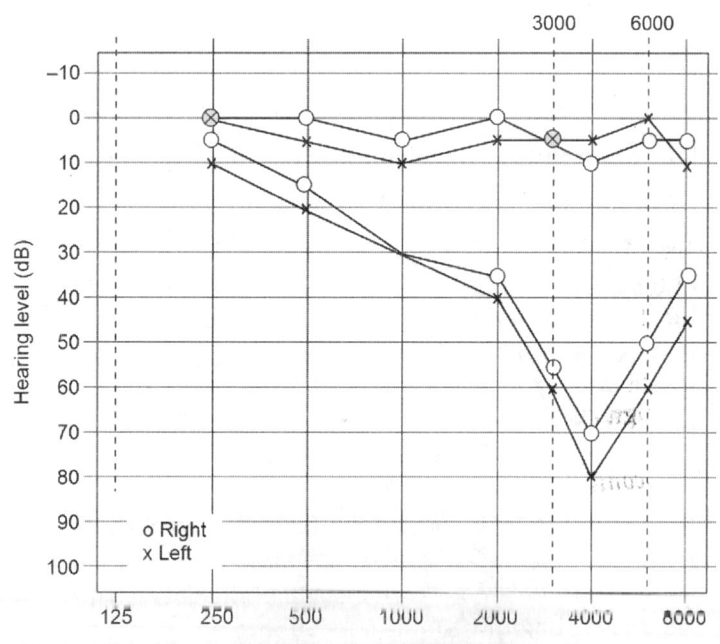

Fig. 7.3: Audiometry: Normal and NIHL

Chapter

8

Notifiable Occupational Diseases: Pictographs

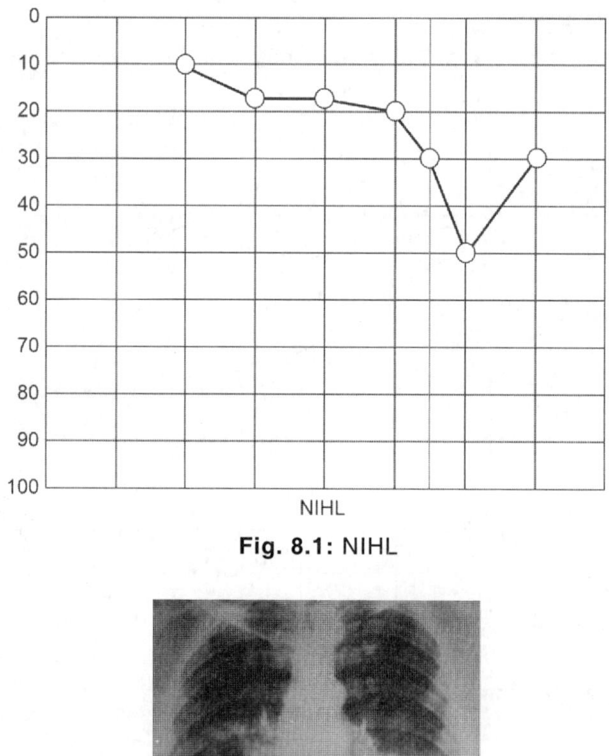

Fig. 8.1: NIHL

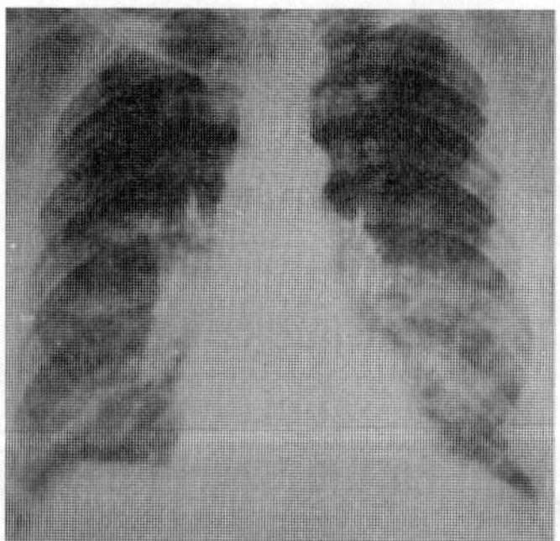

Fig. 8.2: Asbestosis

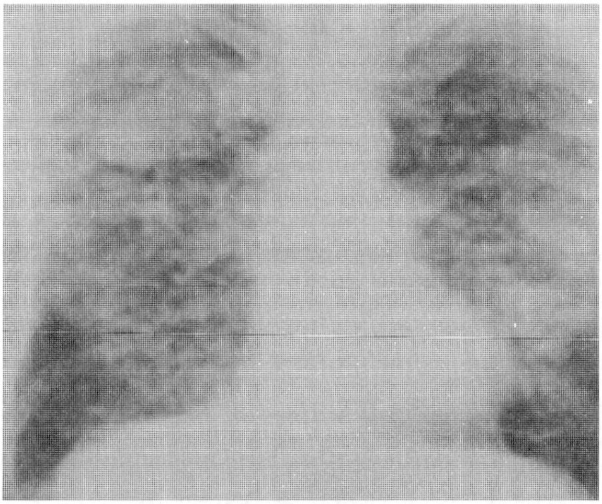

Fig. 8.3: CWP

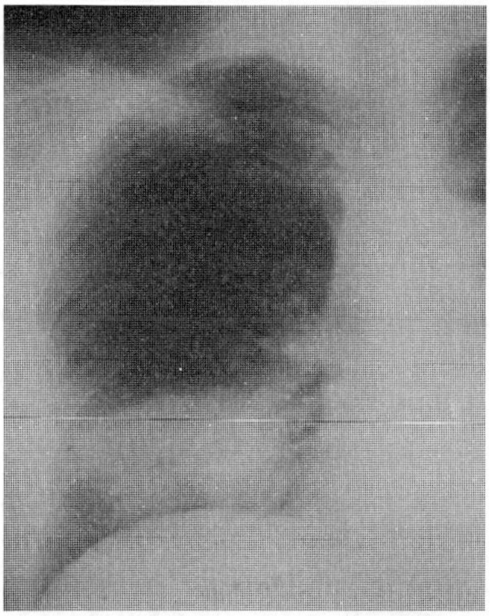

Fig. 8.4: Asbestos lung cancer

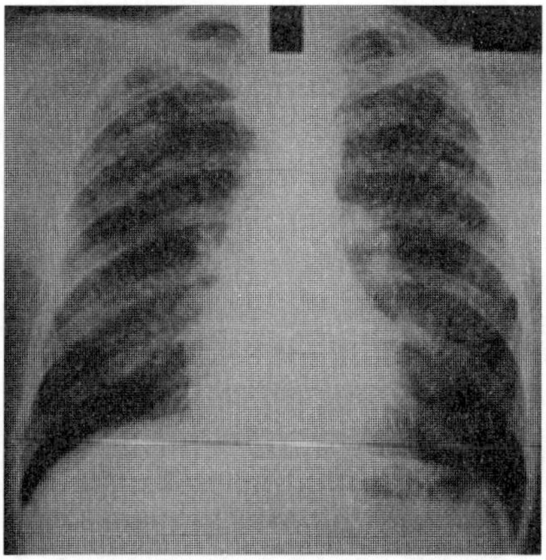

Fig. 8.5: Chronic silicosis

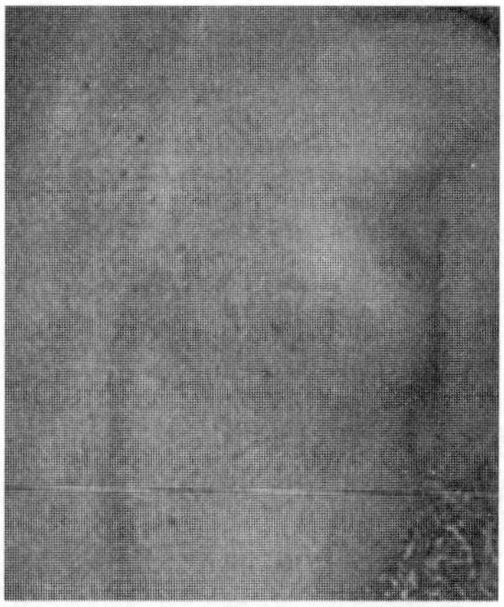

Fig. 8.6: Malignant mesothelioma

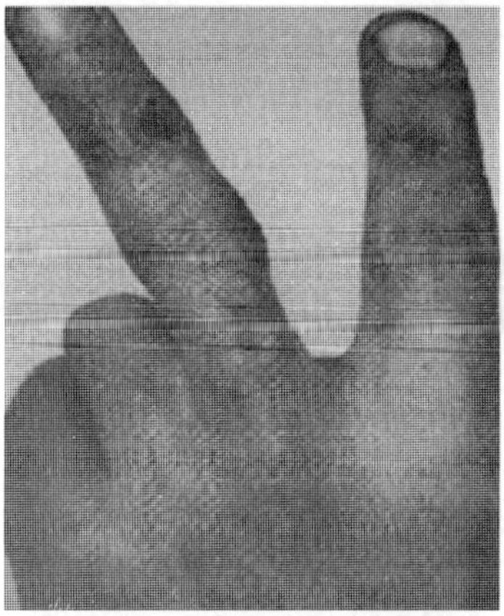

Fig. 8.7: Chrome hole

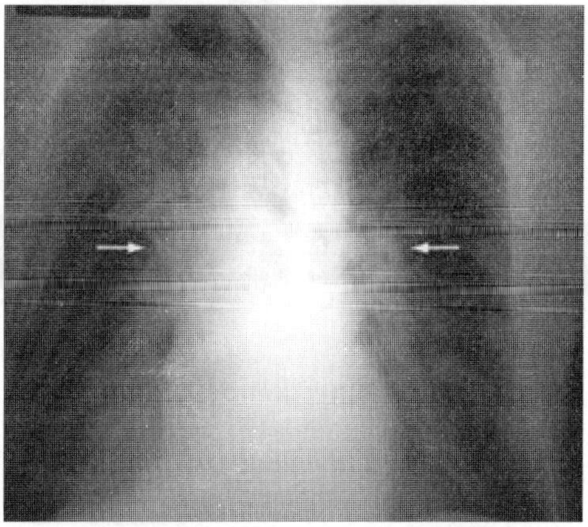

Fig. 8.8: Pulmonary anthrax

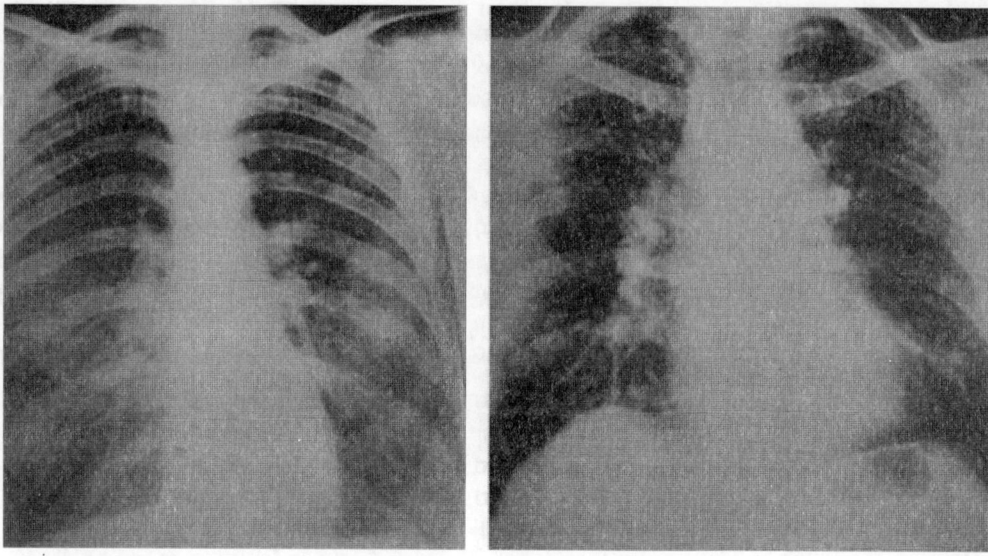

Fig. 8.9: Chronic beryllium disease

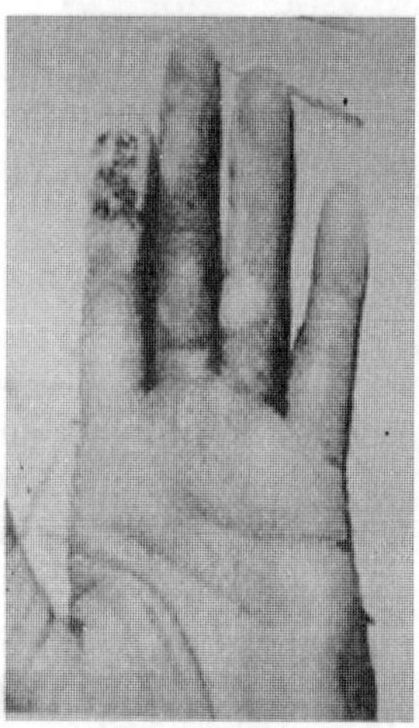

Fig. 8.10: Ionizing burn

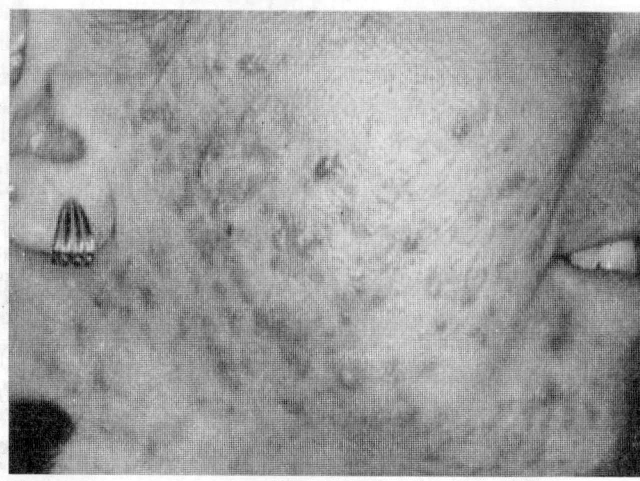

Fig. 8.11: Oil acne

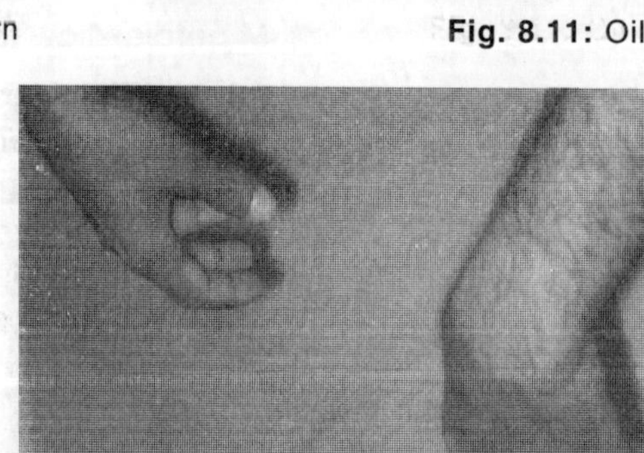

Fig. 8.12: Wrist drop in lead toxicity

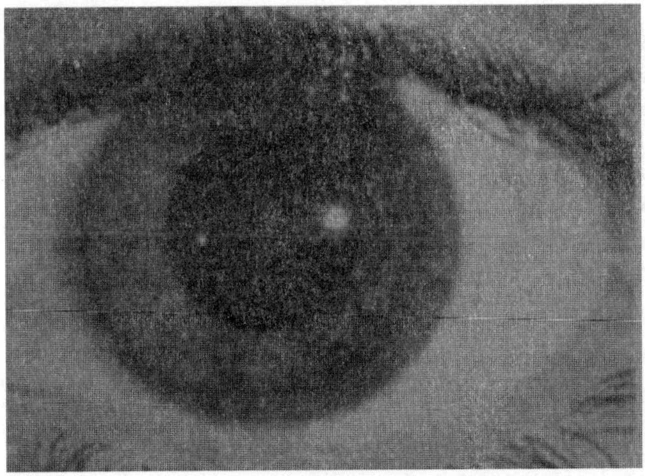

Fig. 8.13: Mercuria lentis

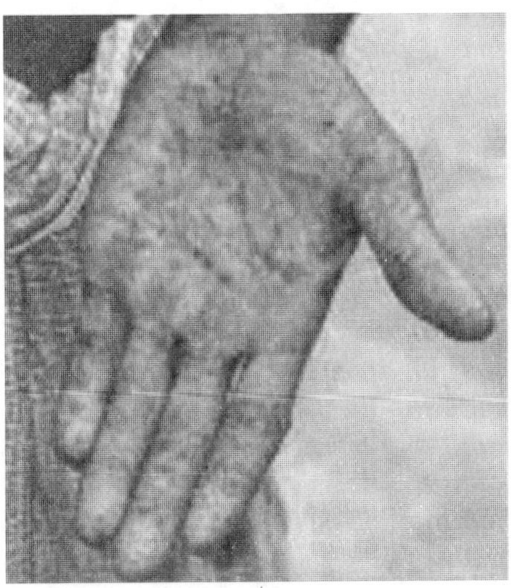

Fig. 8.14: Raindrop pigmentation of arsenic poisoning

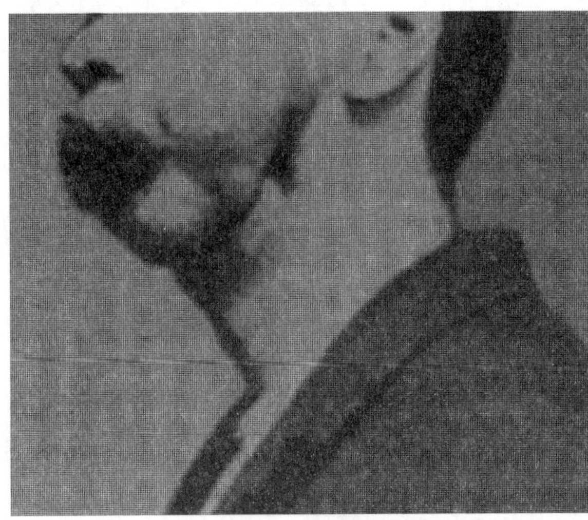

Fig. 8.15: Possy jaw

Chapter

9

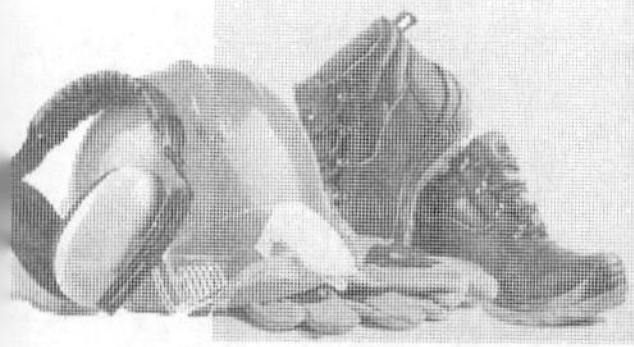

Miscellaneous

IMPLEMENTATION OF NATIONAL POLICY FOR EXCELLENCE IN SAFETY, HEALTH AND ENVIRONMENT (SHE) MANAGEMENT FOR INDUSTRIAL DEVELOPMENT IN INDIA

Industrialization is a global phenomenon and India is no exception. Industrialization is very much needed for economic growth and to face the global challenges. With rapid technological advances in industrial process, newer types of dangers to the life are being increasingly introduced. The management has to play prime role to resolve these issues and restore values through following definite aims:

- To fulfil the commitment towards constitutional requirement
- To comply the statutory requirement
- To run the organization smoothly
- To maximization the profit
- To render accident/illness free service
- To improve its employees
- To create new employment opportunity
- To serve the society
- To enrich the nation.

The constitutional requirement for the management of the industry is to implement the concerned articles of "Directive Principles of State Policy" like:

Article 39: Directs for securing the health and strength of employees, men and women, that the tender age of children is not abused, that citizens are not forced by economic necessity to enter avocations unsuited to their age or strength.

Article 43A: States that the government shall take steps, by suitable legislation or in any other way, to secure the participation of employee in the management of undertakings, establishments or other organizations.

Article 24: Directs for ensuring that no child below 14 years is employed to work in any factory or mine or engaged in any other hazardous employment.

On the basis of these Directive Principles and International Instruments, the Government of India declared National Policy on "Safety, Health and Environment at Workplace" duly approved by the Union Cabinet on 20th February, 2009 in New Delhi during the Indian Labour Conference.

Goal of the National Policy

1. Framing a statutory framework on safety, health and environment (SHE).
2. Developing research and development capability.
3. Improving data collection system on work-related injuries and diseases.
4. Developing and mobilizing required technical OSHE manpower.
5. OSHE as integral component in every operation and in other relevant national policy.

Objective of National Policy

1. Continuous reduction in the incidence of work-related fatal and non-fatal injuries, occupational diseases.
2. Improve coverage of work-related injuries, fatalities and diseases and provide for a more comprehensive data base.
3. Continuous enhancement of community awareness.
4. Continuous increase community expectation of workplace health and safety standard.
5. Improving SHE at workplace by creation of 'green jobs'.

Action Program

1. Enforcement by the State Enforcement Authority.
2. National standard by BIS and other concerned authority.
3. Compliance of safety statutes and standards by the industry.
4. Awareness program by the government, industries and OSH stakeholders.
5. Research and development by all concerned.
6. Data collection and formation of data bank.
7. Review of OSH status through audits, studies and surveys.
8. Review/update SHE policies at workplace.

Accident scenario in industries in India (standard reference)					
Type of Accident	*Year*				
	2007	2008	2009	2010	2011
Fatal	1464	1369	1509	1459	1433
Non-fatal	32526	32570	31584	30046	28402

INDUSTRIAL SAFETY, HEALTH AND HYGIENE

The principles, which need to state the basic philosophy that will guide future efforts in safety, may include something similar to the following:

1. Safety must be at least equal to all other business activities.
2. Management must demonstrate a clear commitment to safety.
3. Safety improvement requires continuous change.
4. Management must provide the resources for continuous improvement.

Resources provided by management may include, but are not limited to, the following:

1. Safety and health team.
2. Training and education materials, including instructors.
3. Time for training and education.

4. Personal protective equipment.
5. Technology review for training needs.
6. Funds to correct recognized hazards.

Some basic ingredients are needed for the development of an effective safety and health plan for continuous improvement. Safety and health programs may vary as to the implementation of each ingredient, but programs should include:

1. Defined objectives, goals, and measurements.
2. Organizational commitment.
3. Evaluation of hazards and the causes of hazards.
4. Facility and equipment design.
5. Effective communication, training, and educational programs.
6. Corrective action programs and performance audit.

Some of the methods that can be used to review the workplace for existing hazards:

1. Utilizing safety and health professionals for periodic audits.
2. Training everyone to recognize known hazards.
3. Performing periodic inspections of equipment and work areas.
4. Performing process analyses for potential problems.
5. Investigating all accidents with potential to cause accidents.
6. Organizing committees to review specific problems.

Industrial hygiene is devoted to the anticipation, recognition, evaluation, and control of environmental factors or stresses arising in or from the workplace, which can cause sickness, impaired health and well-being, or significant discomfort among workers or among citizens of the community. The role of industrial hygienist in the work setting is to provide expertise in identifying health hazards, using accepted instrumentation and methodologies to evaluate their magnitude and to provide advice on implementation of control measures. One aspect of that role is to provide information to the occupational health practitioners on the hazards posed by work processes. An effective industrial hygiene program must be proactive in recognizing potential hazards and setting up sound programs that reduce exposure hazards.

OCCUPATIONAL HEALTH CARE MANAGEMENT SYSTEM

Occupational health care management system is now classified into two levels: International and National.

INTERNATIONAL LEVEL

Some of the international organizations dealing with occupational health:

1. *World Health Organization (WHO)*: World Health Organization is a specialized, non-political, health agency of the United Nations with headquarters at Geneva. The constitution came into force on 7th April, 1948 which is celebrated every year as "World Health Day". The works of WHO are:
   a. Prevention and control of specific diseases.
   b. Development of comprehensive health services.
   c. Family health.
   d. Environmental health.

e. Health statistics.
f. Biomedical research.
g. Health literature and information
h. Cooperation with other organizations.

International Labour Organization (ILO)

The International Labour Organization was established in 1919 with Headquarter at Geneva, Switzerland. The purposes of ILO are:

a. To contribute to the establishment of lasting peace by promoting social justice.
b. To improve, through international action, labour conditions and living standards.
c. To promote economic and social stability. There is a close collaboration between ILO and WHO in the field of health and labour

The United Nations Development Programme (UNDP)

The United Nations Development Programme was established in 1966. It is the main source of funds for technical assistance. The basic objective of UNDP is to help poorer nations develop their human and natural resources more fully. It covers every economic and social sector like agricultural, industry, education, science, health, and social welfare.

The Food and Agricultural Organization (FAO)

The Food and Agricultural Organization was formed in 1945 with Headquarter at Rome. The joint WHO/FAO expert Committee has provided many cooperative activities like nutrition survey, research on brucellosis and other zoonoses.

World Bank

It was established with the purpose of helping less developed countries raise their living standards. Health and environmental components have been added to many projects.

The Colombo Plan

At a meeting of the Commonwealth Foreign Ministers at Colombo in January, 1950, a programme was drawn up for cooperative economic development in south and south-east Asia. Membership comprises 20 developing countries within the region and 6 non-regional members: Australia, Canada, Japan, New Zealand, UK, and USA. The bulk of Colombo Plan assistance goes into industrial and agricultural development but some support has also been given to the health promotion. All India Institute of Medical Science at New Delhi was established with the financial assistance from New Zealand.

Rockefeller Foundation

It is a philanthropic organization chartered in 1913 and endowed by Mr. John D. Rockefeller. Its purpose is to promote the well-being of mankind throughout the world. All India Institute of Hygiene and Public Health, Kolkata, was established by this foundation.

International Red Cross

It was founded by Henry Dunant, a young Swiss businessman in 1859. It has many activities like disaster services, first-aid and nursing, health education, etc.

The International Commission on Occupational Health (ICOH)

In 1902, Dr. De Cristoforis, an Italian senator and the head of the Department of Education of the city of Milan, proposed holding an international congress on occupational diseases in celebration of the opening of the Simplon tunnel and, specifically, in commemoration of the 10,000 miners who had died of ankylostomiasis during the construction of the St. Gotthard tunnel. The congress was delayed until 1906; but when it was finally held in Milanin June of that year, the International Permanent Commission on Occupational Medicine was founded with the intend to organize an international congress every third year and to exchange ideas and experiences among leading scientists in occupational medicine. Dr. De Cristoforis was elected the first president of the commission. The adoption of the new membership policy prompted a change of name in 1957. The name was changed to the Permanent Commission and International Association of Occupational Health. This rather awkward name was shortened in 1984 to the International Commission on Occupational Health (ICOH) in connection with a thorough revision of its constitution and by-laws. According to its constitution, ICOH is an international nongovernmental scientific society whose aim is to foster the scientific progress, knowledge, and development of occupational health in all its aspects. The professional distribution of ICOH's members is wide and includes physicians, occupational hygienists, occupational health nurses, safety engineers, psychologists, chemists, ergonomists, statisticians, social scientists, and physiotherapists. Being recognized by the United Nations as a 'nongovernmental organization', ICOH keeps a close working relationship with the World Health Organization (WHO), the International Labour Organization (ILO), and other U.N. bodies, as well as with the commission for European Communities and the International Social Security Association.

NATIONAL LEVEL (IN INDIA)

Occupational health care systems in India are operating at the following three tier systems.

Central Government Level

1. *Directorate General of Factory Advice Service and Labour Institutes (DGFASLI) under Ministry of Labour and Employment, Government of India with Head Office in Mumbai:* Directorate General Factory Advice Service and Labour Institutes (DGFASLI), formerly known as Chief Adviser of Factories, was set up in 1945 at Delhi. The DGFASLI was set up with the objective of advising the Central and the State Governments on administration of the Factories Act, 1948 and liaising with factories inspection services in the States. The office was subsequently shifted to Mumbai in 1966. The DGFASLI is an Attached Office of the Ministry of Labour & Employment, Government of India and serves as a technical arm to assist the Ministry in formulating national policies on occupational safety and health in factories and Docks. It also advises factories on various issues concerning safety, health, efficiency and well-being of the persons at workplace. DGFASLI is a multidisciplinary organization comprising of Occupational Safety Engineers, Occupational Health Doctors, Industrial Hygienists, Industrial Psychologists and Industrial physiologists. DGFASLI organization comprises of the Headquarter and Central Labour Institute located at Mumbai and four Regional Labour Institute at Chennai, Kanpur, Kolkata and Faridabad; and eleven Inspectorates of Dock Safety at Chennai, Cochin, JNPT Navi Mumbai, Kandla, Kolkata, Mormugao, Mumbai, New Mangalore, Paradip, Tuticorin and Visakhapatnam.

2. *Directorate General of Mines Safety (DGMS) under Ministry of Labour and Employment, Government of India with head office at Dhanbad:* In 1895, the Government of India initiated steps to frame legislative measures for safety of workmen in mines. In 1897, first major disaster in mining hit the Kolar Goldfields killing 52 persons, to be soon followed by the Khost Coal Mine disaster in Baluchistan (now in Pakistan) killing 47 persons. The disaster hastened the process of formulation of safety laws and the first Mines Act was enacted in 1901. With further experience, this Act was superseded by the Indian Mines Act, 1923, which was again replaced by the present Mines Act, 1952. This Act came into force on the 1st July 1952. Major changes were incorporated in this Act in the years 1959 and 1983. The Mines Act, 1952 applies to mines of all minerals within the country including the offshore mines within the limits of territorial water. For administering the provisions of the Indian Mines Act, 1901, the Government of India set up a "Bureau of Mines Inspection and Quot"; on the 7th January 1902 with headquarters at Calcutta. The name of the organization was changed to Department of Mines in 1904 and its headquarters shifted to Dhanbad in 1908. On 1.1.1960, the organization was renamed as "Office of the Chief Inspector of Mines". Since 1.5.1967, the office has been re-designated as Directorate General of Mines Safety (DGMS in short). Directorate General of Mines Safety, DGMS in short, is the Regulatory Agency under the Ministry of Labour and Employment, Government of India in matters pertaining to occupational safety, health and welfare of persons employed in mines (coal, metalliferous and oil-mines). Mines Safety (DGMS), under the Union Ministry of Labour and Employment. Apart from administering the Mines Act and the subordinate legislation thereunder, DGMS also administers a few other allied legislations, including the Indian Electricity Act. The organization has its headquarters at Dhanbad (Jharkhand) and is headed by Director General of Mines Safety. At the headquarter, the Director General is assisted by specialist staff-officers in mining, electrical and mechanical, occupational health, law, survey, statistics, administration and accounts disciplines. The headquarters has also a technical library and S&T laboratories as a back-up support to the organization. Due to the nature of work performed by the officers of DGMS, the Government of India declared the organization as S&T Institution" on the recommendation of Science and Technology Department of Government of India, in November 1987. The Vision of DGMS is to attain risk and hazard free conditions of work and welfare of persons employed in mines and the mission is to identify and reduce risk of accidents and diseases in and around the mine through: Development of suitable legislation, rules, regulations, standards and guidelines; Adequate measures to ensure compliance and Awareness initiatives to inculcate safety and health culture amongst work-persons and stakeholders.
3. *Employee State Insurance Corporation (ESIC) under Ministry of Labour and Employment, Government of India*: Employee's State Insurance Corporation is a self-financing social security and health insurance scheme for Indian workers. This fund is managed by the Employees' State Insurance Corporation (ESIC) according to rules and regulations stipulated there in the ESI Act 1948.
4. *National Institute of Occupational Health (NIOH) under Indian Council of Medical Research, Ministry of Health and Family Welfare, Government of India with head office in Ahmedabad:* National Institute of Occupational Health is a premier public health institute, which was established in 1966 as Occupational Health Research Institute (OHRI), taking 2 rooms at BJ Medical College, Ahmedabad. The OHRI was later renamed as "National Institute of Occupational Health" (NIOH) in 1970 and was moved to its present premises. Since then, till now, NIOH has been working continuously through its main as well its regional

centers. The primary responsibility of NIOH is to support the national policy makers for adopting an appropriate policy in the field of occupational health, based on felt needs of our country. This is done through multidisciplinary research, capacity building and technological development.

5. *Industrial Toxicology Research Centre (ITRC) under CSIR, Government of India with Head Office at Lucknow*: Industrial Toxicology Research Centre (ITRC), Lucknow, a constituent laboratory of Council of Scientific and Industrial Research (CSIR) is dedicated to provide health safeguards to industrial and agricultural workers through its rich knowledge base. ITRC was established in 1965. The institute organises outreach programs and public awareness camps to communicate the knowledge widely so that the information is put to practical use by regulators, policy makers and other scientists in industry, government and academies. Following services are being rendered to industries, public sector undertakings and Government R&D organizations:
   a. *Health survey*: Epidemiological surveys/studies on occupational diseases in industrial workers and the required remedial measures.
   b. *Environmental monitoring*: Air and water quality monitoring studies for industries as well as government organisations are undertaken.
   c. *Analytical services*: Analysis of metal, pesticides, polycyclic aromatic hydrocarbons, etc. in various samples including human tissues are undertaken with latest techniques.
   d. *Safety evaluation of products*: Agrochemicals, dyes, food additives, plastics and polymers, petrochemicals, cosmetics, detergents, organic and mineral fibers and particulate material are tested for their safety as per requirement of the registration authorities.
   e. *Food adulterants*: The center plays a major role in providing services to both private and government sector for the identification and safety of food adulterants.
   f. *Ecotoxicological impact assessment*.
   g. *Toxicity of chemicals*: Studies on chemicals are undertaken using validated test systems to assess their: Mutagenicity and carcinogenicity, genotoxicity, LD_{50}, phytotoxicity, photo oxidative damage, microbial conversion of liquid wastes to useful/utilizable commodities.
   h. *Screening of compounds*: Using *in vivo* and rapid *in vitro* test systems, compounds are screened for various properties such as screening of the psychoactive compounds and neurotoxicants with the help of neurotransmitter receptor binding assays.
   i. *Safety evaluation of industrial/environmental chemicals*: ITRC has been offering its services for the assessment and abatement of problems in occupational and environmental toxicology on sponsored basis.
6. *All India Institute of Hygiene and Public Health (AIIH&PH) under Ministry of Health and Family Welfare, Government of India with Head Office in Kolkata:* All India Institute of Hygiene and Public Health (AIIH&PH) is a pioneering Indian Institute for Research and Training in Public Health and Allied Sciences in Kolkata. It was established on 30 December, 1932 with assistance from the Rockefeller Foundation. It functions under Director General of Health Services, New Delhi, Ministry of Health and Family Welfare, Government of India.
7. *National Environmental Engineering Research Institute under CSIR, Government of India with head office at Nagpur:* The CSIR-National Environmental Engineering Research Institute (CSIR-NEERI) is a research institute created and funded by Government of India. It was established in Nagpur in 1958 with focus on water supply, sewage disposal,

communicable diseases and to some extent on industrial pollution and occupational diseases found common in post-independent India. NEERI is a pioneer laboratory in the field of environmental science and engineering and part of Council of Scientific and Industrial Research (CSIR). NEERI has five zonal laboratories at Chennai, Delhi, Hyderabad, Kolkata and Mumbai. NEERI falls under the Ministry of Science and Technology, Government of India.

8. *Central Pollution Control Board (CPCB) under Ministry of Environment and Forest, Government of India.*
9. *National Institute of Miners' Health under Ministry of Mines, Government of India with head office at Nagpur*: National Institute of Miners' Health, Nagpur (NIMH) is an autonomous institute established in 1990 under Ministry of Mines, Government of India with the objective of promotion of occupational health and prevention of occupational diseases among the workers employed in mining and mineral based industries. The institute is engaged in research and developmental activities relating to occupational health, workplace monitoring, etc. in mines and mineral based industries. The institute also conducts training program for development of manpower in these fields. Very recently, this organization has been merged with the National Institute of Occupational Health (NIOH), Ahmedabad.
10. *National Safety Council (NSC), Autonomous Body under Ministry of Labour and Employment, Government of India with Head Office in Navi Mumbai.*
11. *Central Mining and Research Station under CSIR, Government of India at Cuttack, Dhanbad, Jamshedpur & Bhavnagar.*
12. *All Central Government Medical College and Hospitals.*
13. *Indian Institute of Technology, Kanpur, UP.*
14. *Indian Association of Occupational Health (IAOH), a Non-Government Organization (NGO)*: Indian Association of Occupational Health (IAOH) was founded in 1948 by group of enlightened Industrial Physicians to create awareness about occupational diseases in India and to suggest preventive measures. It is affiliated to International Commission on Occupational Health (ICOH) and American Industrial Hygiene Association. This is the apex National Professional Non-Government Society in the field of occupational health.
15. *Indian Medical Association (IMA), a Non-Governmental Organization (NGO).*

State Government Level

a. Inspectorate of Factories and Boilers/Directorate of Industrial Safety and Health (DISH), Department of Labour.
b. Employee State Insurance (ESI), Department of Labour.
c. State Pollution Control Board.
d. Certifying Surgeon.
e. Medical College and Hospitals under State Government
f. Non-Governmental Organizations (NGOs).

Unit Level (Factory Level)

a. Occupational Health Centre/First-aid Centre.
b. Industrial Hospital.
c. Local Governmental and Private health care units.
d. Factory Medical Officers and Occupational Health Nurses.

e. Private Practitioners or Registered Medical Practitioners (RMO).
f. First-Aid Box in Industry.

HEALTH PROMOTION PROGRAMS IN INDUSTRY

Screening

Screening examinations are commonly used as entry points for health promotion programs. The components of the examination should be assessed for sensitivity and specificity, has a reasonable cost, follow WHO criteria, be directly relevant to proposed activities, and address a condition with a high enough prevalence in the population that there is a reasonable yield.

Hypertension and Cholesterol Control

High blood pressure and high blood cholesterol levels are important risks for cardiovascular disease. Worksite screening programs have proved successful in the detection of these conditions and initiation of non-pharmacologic therapy, stress management, smoking cessation, weight reduction and fitness. These interventions have been shown to reduce total serum cholesterol, low-density lipoproteins (LDL) and blood pressure to varying degrees. If non-pharmacologic management does not completely control blood pressure or cholesterol, referral for further diagnostic evaluation and pharmacologic therapy can be made.

Fitness

Improved fitness is thought to increase attendance, performance and productivity, reduce stress and depression, help control weight, substance use, and blood sugar, increase high-density lipoprotein (HDL) levels, and decrease the risk of cardiovascular disease.

Smoking Control

The most effective smoking control programs are multifaceted and include self-help materials, smoking cessation programs, and a smoke-free environment. Smoke-free workplace policies emphasize protection of all employees' health including avoidance of allergic and irritant effects as well as the more serious effects of passive smoke inhalation.

Other Substance Abuse Control

As with smoking, programs to deal with other addictive behaviors should be comprehensive. Key elements include a drug-free workplace policy and preventive education to deal with co-dependency, addictive personalities, and the social and physical effects of substance use and abuse on employees and their families. Employee-assistance programs are important to provide screening and early intervention. Drug-free workplace policies should clearly establish a workplace environment which does not permit the use of mind- or mood-altering substances in the interest of safety, courtesy, equal workload, and productivity.

Employee-Assistance Programs

While employee-assistance programs have provided secondary rather than primary prevention, they are now merging with health-promotion programs, since the behavior-change techniques and systems orientation that employee-assistance programs use are quite effective for other health-related behaviors in addition to substance abuse and mental disorders.

Stress Management

The stress reaction is a neuroendocrine response to the perception of threat from physical, emotional, and organizational stressors. As stress accumulates without reversal, there are longer-term effects such as immune system compromise, muscle tension and pain, and various behavioral consequences such as explosive behavior and poor decision-making. Periodic (e.g. twice daily) triggering of the alpha state (a type of brain wave rhythm) for periods of 20 minutes or longer allows the body to reset various muscular servomechanisms to lower levels and reverse other effects of stress. There are a number of well-accepted techniques for eliciting this response, including the "relaxation response", progressive muscular relaxation, some forms of stretching, various meditation techniques, and creative visualization. Another widely used stress management technique is regular aerobic exercise. Exercise apparently acts by reducing muscular tension, increasing endorphin levels, possibly by triggering the alpha state through rhythmic motion (runner's high), and by reducing levels of circulating catecholamines and steroids which accumulate as a result of a stress reaction.

Nutrition Programs

Nutrition program should be aimed at the widest range of problems which pose the greatest pooled risk to the employee population.

Medical Self-care Programs and Wise-use Education

In many corporate benefits programs, a significant amount of resources are expended on "ill-defined complaints"—vague symptoms for which employees and dependents seek medical advice. Self-care and wise-use education can result in a 17–35% decrease in health care costs in these cases. A number of approaches can be taken, ranging from provision of newsletters, pamphlets, and books to classes or 'point-of-need' advice services.

AIDS Education

These activities provide objective information to employees and dependents for two reasons: to enable people to protect themselves from the spread of AIDS, and to reduce the inappropriate fear of persons who carry the human immunodeficiency virus (HIV).

MATERIAL SAFETY DATA SHEET (MSDS)

1. Chemical manufacturers and importers are required to obtain or develop a material safety data sheet for each hazardous chemical they produce or import. Distributors are responsible for ensuring that their customers are provided a copy of these MSDSs. Employers must have an MSDS for each hazardous chemical which they use. Employers may rely on the information received from their suppliers.
2. Each material safety data sheet shall be in English (although the employer may maintain copies in other languages as well), and shall obtain at least the following information:
   i. The identity used on the label (except in some trade secret):
      a. If the hazardous chemical is a single substance, its chemical and common name(s).
      b. If the hazardous chemical is a mixture which has been tested as a whole to determine its hazards, the chemical and common name(s) of the ingredients which contribute to these known hazards, and the common name(s) of the mixture itself.

c. If the hazardous chemical is a mixture which has not been tested as a whole:
   - The chemical and common name(s) of all ingredients which have been determined to be health hazards, and which comprise 1% or greater of the composition, except that chemical identified as carcinogen shall be listed if the concentrations are 0.1% or greater.
   - The chemical and common name(s) of all ingredients which have been determined to be health hazards, and which comprise <1% (0.1% for carcinogens) of the mixture, if there is evidence that the ingredient(s) could be released from the mixture in concentrations which would exceed an established OSHA permissible exposure limit or ACGIH threshold limit value (TLV), or could present a health risk to employees.
   - The chemical and common name(s) of all ingredients which have been determined to present a physical hazard when present in the mixture.

ii. Physical and chemical characteristics of the hazardous chemical (such as vapor pressure, flash point).

iii. The physical hazardous of the hazardous chemical, including the potential of for fire, explosion, and reactivity.

iv. The health hazards of the hazardous chemical, including signs and symptoms of exposure, and any medical conditions which are generally recognized as being aggravated by exposure to the chemical.

v. The primary route(s) of entry.

vi. The OSHA permissible exposure limit, ACGIH threshold limit value (TLV) and any other exposure limit used or recommended by the chemical manufacturer, importer, or employer preparing the material safety data sheet, where available.

vii. Whether the hazardous chemical is listed in the National Toxicology Programme (NTP) Annual Report on carcinogens (latest edition) or has been found to be a potential carcinogen in the International Agency for Research on Cancer (IARC) Monographs (latest edition), or by OSHA.

viii. Any generally applicable precautions for safe handling and use which are known to the chemical manufacturer, importer, or employer preparing MSDS, including appropriate hygienic practices, protective measures during repair and maintenance of contaminated equipment, and procedures for clean-up of spills and leaks.

ix. Any generally applicable control measures which are known to the chemical manufacturer, importer, or employer preparing MSDS, such as appropriate engineering controls, work practices, or personal protective equipment (PPE).

x. Emergency and first aid procedures.

xi. The date of preparation of MSDS or the last change to it.

xii. The name, address and telephone number of the chemical manufacturer, importer, employer, or other responsible party preparing or distributing the MSDS who can provide additional information on the hazardous chemical and appropriate emergency procedures, if necessary.

3. If no relevant information is found for any given category on the material safety data sheet, the chemical manufacturer, importer, or employer preparing MSDS shall make it to indicate that no applicable information was found.
4. Where complex mixture has similar hazards and contents (i.e. the chemical ingredients are essentially the same, but the specific composition varies from mixture to mixture), the

chemical manufacturer, importer, or employer may prepare one MSDS to apply to all of these similar mixtures.

5. The chemical manufacturer, importer, or employer preparing MSDS shall ensure that the information recorded accurately reflects the scientific evidence used in making the hazard determination. If the chemical manufacturer, importer, or employer preparing MSDS becomes newly aware of any significant information regarding the hazards of the chemical or ways to protect against the hazards, this new information shall be added to the material safety data sheet, within 3 months. If the chemical is not currently being produced or imported the chemical manufacturer, importer, or employer shall add the information to the MSDS before the chemical is introduced into the workplace again.
6. i. Chemical manufacturers or importers shall ensure that distributors and employers are provided an appropriate MSDS with their initial shipment after a material safety data sheet is updated.
   ii. The chemical manufacturers or importers shall either provide MSDS with the shipped containers or send them to the distributor or employer prior to or at the time of the shipment.
   iii. If the MSDS is not provided with a shipment that has been labeled as a hazardous chemical, the distributor or employer shall obtain one from the chemical manufactures as soon as possible.
   iv. Chemical manufacturers or importers shall also provide distributors or employers MSDS upon request.
7. i. Distributors shall ensure that MSDSs, and updated information, are provided to other distributors and employers with their initial shipment and with the first shipment after a MSDS is updated.
   ii. The distributors shall either provide MSDSs with shipped containers or send them to other distributor or employer prior to or at the time of shipment.
   iii. Retail distributors selling hazardous chemicals to employers having a commercial account shall provide a MSDS to such employers upon request.
   iv. Wholesale distributors selling hazardous chemical to employers over-the-counter may also provide MSDS upon the request of the employer at the time of over-the-counter purchase.
8. The employer shall maintain the workplace copies of the required MSDSs for each hazardous chemical, and shall ensure that they are readily accessible during each work shift to employees when they are in their work area(s).
9. Where employees must travel between workplaces during a work shift, i.e. their work is carried out at more than one geographical location; the MSDSs may be kept at the primary workplace facility.
10. MSDS may be kept in any form, including operating procedures, and may be designed to cover groups of hazardous chemicals in a work area where it may be more appropriate to address the hazards of a process rather than individual hazardous chemicals.

OCCUPATIONAL HEALTH AND PRODUCTIVITY

Employee health and its effect on productivity are emerging as a critical focus for businesses and occupational health. Employers are realizing that the direct costs of insurance premiums are not what affect the bottom line. The indirect costs of absenteeism and 'presenteeism' (lessened job performance owing to chronic health problems) are also significant drain on company resources. Companies are recognizing that employees are their most important asset and often are not replaced easily. A healthy workforce is now seen as essential to long-term productivity. Companies traditionally believed that high performance was linked primarily to cognitive abilities. However, recent research demonstrates that in order to sustain business growth, employers must be aware of the effect of human health on performance. Employees must have optimal health to maintain optimal productivity. Health care is not only a cost, but it is also an investment in the economic health of the company. Health care costs need to be targeted toward interventions that lessen health risks, decrease the incidence of new diseases, and mitigate the impact of chronic diseases on workers. Measuring the effect of health on productivity is an emerging field. Occupational physicians and nurses understand the workplace and have substantial expertise in disability management. They understand the barriers that may occur before returning an employee back to work and the issues that may delay recovery or affect performance. Occupational physicians and nurses already play roles in workers' compensation disability management, decreasing workers' compensation costs and promoting an early safe return to work. An occupational health specialist is the key player in an integrated health management system. This system should encompass medical programs including return to work, reliance on evidence-based medicine protocol, treating minor non-work-related illness, and using employee assistance programs. There needs to be an internal process to change the work culture to one of total wellness and prevention, including workers' training, the development of information systems to track and report trends, and data analysis to identify areas for opportunity. By using a health and productivity questionnaire, the occupational health professional is able to analyse the health needs of a company. The medical department will know which chronic diseases affect their workplace and to what extent. The physician or nurse will be able to prioritize the programs and determine what consulting and case-management systems will benefit the company most. Working with benefits and human resources, the physician or nurse can help the company to determine which health benefits need strengthening and what services should change based on the chronic health conditions and the medical risk factors of their specific workforce (Fig. 9.1).

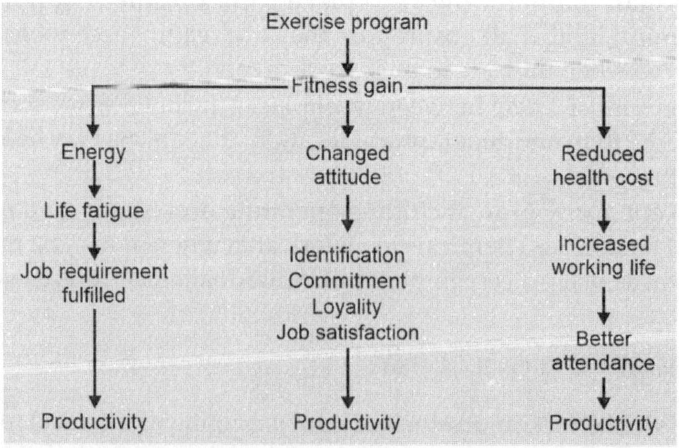

Fig. 9.1: Mechanism of productivity gain from fitness

KAIZEN PHILOSOPHY OF CONTINUOUS IMPROVEMENT

Kaizen is an approach to creating continuous improvement based on the idea that small, ongoing positive changes can reap major improvements. Typically, it is based on cooperation and commitment and stands in contrast to approaches that use radical changes or top-down edicts to achieve transformation. Slow and Steady: Kaizen for 'improvement', or 'change for the better' refers to a philosophy that focuses on continuous improvement of processes in manufacturing, engineering, game development, and business management.

Kaizen is a compound of two Japanese words that together translate as 'good change' or 'improvement', but Kaizen has come to mean 'continuous improvement' through its association with lean methodology. As a broad concept that carries myriad interpretations, it has been adopted in many other industries, including healthcare. Regardless of methodology, in an organizational setting, the successful use of Kaizen rests on gaining support for the approach across the organization, and from the CEO down. Kaizen has its origins in post-World War II Japanese quality circles. These circles or groups of workers focused on preventing defects at Toyota and were developed partly in response to American management and productivity consultants who visited the country, especially W. Edwards Deming, who argued that quality control should be put more directly in the hands of line workers. Kaizen was brought to the West and popularized by Masaaki Imai via his book *Kaizen: The Key to Japan's Competitive Success* in 1986.

Principles of Kaizen

Because executing Kaizen requires enabling the right mindset throughout the company, 10 principles that address the Kaizen mindset are commonly referenced as core to the philosophy. They are:

1. Let go of assumptions.
2. Be proactive about solving problems.
3. Do not accept the status quo.
4. Let go of perfectionism and take an attitude of iterative, adaptive change.
5. Look for solutions as you find mistakes.
6. Create an environment in which everyone feels empowered to contribute.
7. Do not accept the obvious issue; instead, ask 'why' five times to get to the root cause.
8. Call information and opinions from multiple people.
9. Use creativity to find low-cost, small improvements.
10. Never stop improving.

Kaizen Cycle for Continuous Improvement

1. *Get employees involved:* Seek the involvement of employees, including gathering their help in identifying issues and problems. Doing so creates buy-in for change. Often, this is organized as specific groups of individuals charged with gathering and relaying information from a wider group of employees.
2. *Find problems:* Using widespread feedback from all employees, gather a list of problems and potential opportunities. Create a shortlist if there are many issues.
3. *Create a solution:* Encourage employees to offer creative solutions, with all manner of ideas encouraged. Pick a winning solution or solutions from the ideas presented.

4. *Test the solution:* Implement the winning solution chosen above, with everyone participating in the rollout. Create pilot programs or take other small steps to test out the solution.
5. *Analyse the results:* At various intervals, check progress, with specific plans for who will be the point of contact and how best to keep ground-level workers engaged. Determine how successful the change has been.
6. *Standardize:* If results are positive, adopt the solution throughout the organization.
7. *Repeat:* These seven steps should be repeated on an ongoing basis, with new solutions tested where appropriate or new lists of problems tackled.

Advantages

1. With its focus on gradual improvement, Kaizen can create a gentler approach to change in contrast to big efforts that may be abandoned due to their tendency to provoke change resistance and abandonment.
2. Kaizen encourages scrutiny of processes so that mistakes and waste can be reduced.
3. Inspection needs are lessened, because errors are reduced.
4. Employee morale grows, because it engenders a sense of value and purposefulness.
5. Teamwork increases as employees think beyond the specific issues of their department.
6. Client focus increases as customer requirements awareness is raised.
7. Systems are in place to ensure improvements are encouraged both short- and long-term.

Disadvantages

1. Companies with cultures of territorialism and closed communication may first need to focus on cultural changes to create a receptive environment.
2. Short-term Kaizen events may create a burst of excitement that is shallow and short-lived and, therefore, gets abandoned before long.

Bibliography

1. Akron OH. American Industrial Hygiene Association (AIHA), 1975. Heating and Cooling of Man in Industry, 2nd ed.
2. American Conference of Governmental Industrial Hygienists: Particle size-selective sampling in the workplace. Cinncinnati, 1984.
3. American Conference of Governmental Industrial Hygienists (ACGIH). 1990. Documentation of Threshold Limit values and Biological Exposure Indices. 6th ed. Cincinnati.
4. American Conference of Governmental Industrial Hygienists (ACGIH). 199, 1992-93. Documentation of Threshold Limit values and Biological Exposure Indices. 6th ed. Cincinnati.
5. American National Standards Institute, New York: Criteria for background noise in the audiometer room.
6. Antero Aitio, Vesa Riihimaki, Jyrki Liesivuori, Jorma Jarvisalo, Sven Hernberg. Biological Monitoring.
7. Battigelli MC. Determination of fitness to work.
8. Benoit N. Metal dusts and fumes.
9. Bodaghpoura S, Biglari N Joob, Ahmadib S. A review on the existence of chrome in cement and environmental remedies to control its effects. punlished in International Journal of Geology: 2012; 2(6).
10. Cailliet R. Low Back Pain Syndrome. 2nd Edition. 1968, Philadelphia: FA Davis Co.
11. Carl Zenz, O Bruce Dickerson, Edward P Horvath Jr. Occupational Medicine. 3rd Edition.
12. Chicago IL. National Safety Council. 1985. Pocket Guide to Heat Stress.
13. Crofton and Douglas. Respiratory Diseases: 5th Edition.
14. Datta SR , Chatterjee BB, Roy BN. An Improved Simple Exercise Test for Evaluation of Physical Fitness.
15. Davidson's Principles and Practice of Medicine: Edited by Brian R Walker, Nicki R Colledge, Stuart H Ralston, Ian D Penman: 22nd Edition.
16. Dickerson OB, Walter E Baker. Practical Ergonomics and work with Video Display Terminals.
17. Dudley B. Trauma and Emergencies in the Workplace: General Principles.
18. Environmental Medicine: Integrating a Missing Element into Medical Education (1995), Chapter: Case Study 52: Behavioral and audiologic Manifestations of Noise-Induced Hearing Loss.
19. Franklin T. Hoaglund. Musculoskeletal Injuries:
20. Haldar SK. Occupational and Industrial Health, 1st Edition.
21. Harrison's Principles of Internal Medicine, 17th Edition.
22. Heat Stress: OSHA Technical Manual (OTM), Section III: Chapter IV.
23. Hope S Rugo. Occupational Cancer.
24. Howard E, Oakley N. Heat and Cold.
25. Hunter's Diseases of Occupations. Edited by Peter J Baxter, Tar-Ching AW, Anne Cockcroft, Paul Durrington and J Malcolm Harrington (10th Edition).
26. Jos V, Frederieke S. Occupational back pain.
27. Joseph L. Current Occupational and Environmental Medicine. 4th Edition
28. Joseph L. Occupational and Environmental Medicine. 4th Edition.
29. National Institute of Occupational Safety and Health (NIOSH): Standards for Occupational Exposure to Hot Environments: Proceedings of a symposium, DHHS (NIOSH) 1985, Publication No. 85-115.
30. Occupational Lung Diseases: Prevention and Control: International Labour Office, Geneva: Occupational Safety and Health Series (67).
31. OSHA Technical Manual: TED 01-00-015: February 11, 2014, Section II: Chapter 1–3.
32. Park K. Preventive and Social Medicine, 23rd Edition.
33. Particle size-selective sampling in the workplace. Ann Am Conf Govt Ind Hyg, 1884, 11:23–100.

34. Performance consideration for size-selective samplers (revised), Ann Am Conf Govt Ind Hyg (in press).
35. Petrus C Schutte, Carl Zenz. Physical Work and Heat Stress.
36. Raymond W Parkes. Occupational Lung Disorders: 3rd Edition.
37. Rofl H, Walter R. Fatigue and Recovery.
38. Schedule XXIV of Indian Factories Act, 1948, operation involving high noise (Model Factories Rules 120 under Section 87).
39. Snook SH. Approaches to the control of back pain in industry: Job design, job placement and education/ training. Occupational Medicine. 1988; 3:45–59.
40. Stuart A Lavy. Introduction to Occupational Pulmonary Diseases.
41. The Indian Factories Act, 1948.
42. The Occupational Safety, Health and Working Condition Code, 2020.
43. "The Workmen's Compensation Act"—A Guide for Activists by Alternative Law Forum.

Index